D1319831

MORE ADVANCE PRAISE FOR
THE AYURVEDA SOLUTION TO TYPE 2 DIABETES

"Dr. Christensen came up with a natural and effective protocol for type 2 diabetes. Simply follow the guidelines and get back your health."
— **Dr. Manisha Kshirsagar, Ayurvedic Physician, Esthetician, author** of *Enchanting Beauty*

"*The Ayurveda Solution to Type 2 Diabetes* approaches type 2 diabetes from a holistic view and opens up new vistas of Ayurvedic insight for both the general reader and for the healthcare professional. The book is very comprehensive and provides a wonderful how-to-do-it approach targeting the individual constitution, diet, and lifestyle."
— **Dr. Rucha Kelkar, Director of Ayurbliss Integrated Wellness Center**

"Read *The Ayurveda Solution to Type 2 Diabetes* for an eloquent understanding of Ayurvedic mind/body medicine. Dr. Jackie Christensen has created an inspiring and complete program to reverse this widespread disease. I recommend it to everyone interested in Ayurveda and natural medicine."
— **Cynthia Copple, Ayurvedic Doctor, Director, Lotus Holistic Health Institute, Co-Founder Mount Madonna Institute College of Ayurveda, author of *Know Your Blueprint***

"Dr. Jackie Christensen brings delight and deep wisdom to *The Ayurveda Solution to Type 2 Diabetes*. Her guidance will help many live with more joy, balance, and radiance."
— **Kelly (Chloë) Spellman, Esalen Massage Therapist**

THE AYURVEDA SOLUTION TO TYPE 2 DIABETES:

A Clinically Proven Approach to Balance Blood Sugar in 12 Weeks

By Jackie Christensen, PhD, MA-Ay
With Pat Crocker

Humanix Books

THE AYURVEDA SOLUTION TO TYPE 2 DIABETES
Copyright © 2021 by Jackie Christensen and Pat Crocker
All rights reserved

Humanix Books, P.O. Box 20989, West Palm Beach, FL 33416, USA
www.humanixbooks.com | info@humanixbooks.com

Humanix Books is a division of Humanix Publishing, LLC. Its trademark, consisting of the words "Humanix Books," is registered in the Patent and Trademark Office and in other countries.

Disclaimer: The information presented in this book is not specific medical advice for any individual and should not substitute medical advice from a health professional. If you have (or think you may have) a medical problem, speak to your doctor or a health professional immediately about your risk and possible treatments. Do not engage in any care or treatment without consulting a medical professional

For a complete bibliography and list of works referenced in The Ayurveda Solution to Type 2 Diabetes, please visit https://www.practiceayurveda.com/.

ISBN: 9-781-63006-179-1 (Hardcover)
ISBN: 9-781-63006-180-7 (E-book)

Printed in the United States of America
10 9 8 7 6 5 4 3 2 1

This book is dedicated to the person you will become after reading it,
the person who helped you get there, and the person you are now.

TABLE OF CONTENTS

Chapter 1: What Is Ayurveda and What Can It Do for You?

Vata: The Dosha of Movement 3
Pitta: The Dosha of Metabolism 5
Kapha: The Dosha of Structure 8
Your Constitution 10

Chapter 2: Prameha: The Original Type 2 Diabetes

The Six Stages of Type 2 Diabetes 12
Why Type 2 Diabetes Is Unique to You 15
Types of Diabetes According to Ayurveda 16

Chapter 3: Ayurvedic Treatments for Type 2 Diabetes

Dietary Guidelines 19
Recommended Foods for Type 2 Diabetes 20
Foods to Avoid 27
Upgrade Your Lifestyle 27
Make Major Strides with Walking 28
Proven Workouts for Type 2 Diabetes 30
Formulating Your Exercise Program 31
Stoking Your Brain 33
Get Off the Couch 34
Quality Sleep: Not Just a Dream 35
Three Tools to Silence Stress 37
Herbal Therapies 44
Ayurvedic Detoxification: Panchakarma 50

Chapter 4: The 12-Week Program: Introduction

Program Structure 54
Cultivating Support 54
Creating Your Routine for Success 54
Biometric Goal Setting 55
Self-Monitoring Your Blood Sugar 55

Chapter 5: The 12-Week Program: Starting the
8-Week Constitution and Elimination Diet

Identifying Dietary Guidelines 58
Mindful Eating Awareness 60

Establishing a Daily Routine..61
Walking After Meals 61
Determining Your Maximum Heart Rate 62
Preventing Injuries 63
Discovering Your Constitution 64

Chapter 6: The 12-Week Program: 8-Week
Constitution and Elimination Diet for **Vata**

Vata Food Lists 72
Recipes for Vata..75
Sleep Optimization...86
Vata Daily Schedule..88
Lifestyle Enhancement...89
30-Minute Daily Relaxation Practice 89
Exercise..96
Exercise Journal 98
8-Week Supplement Schedule...98

Chapter 7: The 12-Week Program: 8-Week
Constitution and Elimination Diet for **Pitta**

Pitta Food Lists..101
Recipes for Pitta..104
Sleep Optimization...114
Progressive Muscle Relaxation..115
Lifestyle Enhancement...116
Pitta Daily Schedule 116
30-Minute Daily Relaxation Practice 117
Weekly Exercise...123
Exercise Journal 125
8-Week Supplement Schedule...125

Chapter 8: The 12-Week Program: 8-Week
Constitution and Elimination Diet for **Kapha**

Kapha Food Lists 128
Recipes for Kapha 131
Sleep Optimization...143
Kapha Daily Schedule...144
Lifestyle Enhancement...144
30-Minute Daily Relaxation Practice 145
Daily Relaxation Journal 150
Weekly Exercise...151

Exercise Journal 155
8-Week Supplement Schedule 155

Chapter 9: The 12-Week Program: 1-Week Detox and Restoration

Reasons to Detoxify.. 158
Recognizing Toxicity 159
It's All Connected 161
Detoxification Goals... 162
Detoxification Program Structure.. 162
Detoxification Meal Plan 162
Burning Fat 164
Bodywork Treatments 166
Herbs Before and After Meals: Days 1–5... 168
Sipping Warm Water: Days 1–7 169
Purgative on Day 6 169
1-Week Detox and Restoration for Vata... 170
1-Week Detox and Restoration for Pitta... 172
1-Week Detox and Restoration for Kapha.. 174

Chapter 10: The 12-Week Program: 3-Week
Rebuilding and Reintroduction of Foods

Reintroduction of Foods... 178
Vata 3-Week Food Reintroduction Schedule 179
Pitta 3-Week Food Reintroduction Schedule... 180
Kapha 3-Week Food Reintroduction Schedule 180

Chapter 11: Closing Thoughts

Resources.. 183

Blood Sugar and Food Journal 186

Acknowledgments... 197

About the Authors.. 199

Index 200

CHAPTER 1

WHAT IS AYURVEDA AND WHAT CAN IT DO FOR YOU?

Type 2 diabetes, previously known as non-insulin dependent diabetes or adult-onset diabetes, is one of the most significant public health challenges in the twenty-first century. Experts project that by 2035 this preventable healthcare burden will affect 592 million people worldwide. But there is hope! The future is not predetermined, and health professionals around the world are working hard to identify the root causes of type 2 diabetes. The ancient Indian practice of Ayurveda can inform our modern understanding of diabetes and its treatment. A holistic system of medicine, Ayurveda, was developed in India over 5,000 years ago. The term *Ayurveda* comes from the Sanskrit words *ayur* (life) and *veda* (science or knowledge). *Ayurveda* therefore means "knowledge of life." Ayurveda offers many solutions to the type 2 diabetes riddle. It shines light on the various factors that contribute to this disease, providing dietary guidelines, lifestyle choices, and other unique therapies to combat the disease naturally and without prescription medicines.

The Ayurvedic approach to treating type 2 diabetes is complex. It considers the disease processes, the strength of digestion, the presence of toxins, the actions of the *doshas* (energetic forces—we'll come back to this later), the current state of the body, and the patient's constitution. All these factors play an essential role in the development of type 2 diabetes. Ayurveda views this condition as a metabolic disorder—not one disease, but a syndrome with many interrelated imbalances and disorders. Type 2 diabetes is a multifaceted disease that is unique to each individual and deserves a personalized approach to its prevention and treatment. Ayurveda offers a patient-centered approach. We are all unique in our mind-body type, and Ayurveda focuses on the individuality of the person and the nuances of the imbalance. There is no one-size-fits-all treatment for type 2 diabetes, and Ayurveda is unbeatable in its personalized approach.

Type 2 diabetes is a modern lifestyle disease caused by harmful daily habits and routines, often overlayed on a person's genetic predisposition to the disease. The good news is that, according to numerous studies, 80 to 90 percent of all cases of type 2 diabetes can be prevented by making lifestyle changes, such as cleaning up your diet, reducing sedentary time, and increasing exercise. In this book, I'm going to show you exactly how to make simple, long-lasting changes to improve your life. This approach can not only prevent type 2 diabetes, but it can also reverse it.

The foods and herbs recommended in the Ayurvedic diet for type 2 diabetes work to balance blood glucose, optimize digestion, and reduce the buildup of toxic internal waste such as excess mucus and improperly digested food particles. By rediscovering traditional foods, we can reduce our dependence on genetically modified, chemical-laden foods. And through the introduction of Ayurvedic foods into the Western diet, what we eat can become our medicine. Ayurvedic foods are delicious, powerful agents that help heal the body, and they can be incorporated into a wide variety of meals, making our diet a source of medicinal herbs.

In addition to diet and lifestyle, Ayurveda includes detoxification—an in-depth purification method that plays a pivotal role in Ayurveda's preventive and curative power for type 2 diabetes. The 12-week program described in this book includes diet and lifestyle adjustments as well as home detoxification so that you can experience the depth of this nourishing science of life we call Ayurveda. Throughout this program, you will discover your true nature and transform your lifestyle to one that is beneficial and healing for your mind-body type. Personalized medicine is a new concept in modern healthcare, but it is well-established in the tradition of Ayurveda. Ayurveda recognizes that each person has a unique makeup. Just as we are all unique in our genetics, so we are in our Ayurvedic mind-body type.

Ayurveda describes three dynamic life forces, or *doshas*, which control the functions of the mind and body. These three energetic forces are *vata, pitta,* and *kapha.* When they are in balance, we feel good. However, when they are out of balance, they disrupt the functions of the body.

Modern medicine emphasizes the structure of the body. Ayurveda, on the other hand, focuses on the energies behind that structure—the doshas. Doshas are the underlying energies within the mind and body that control the actions of the body's organs. One dosha is not better than the rest; we need all three for the mind and body to operate. What makes us unique is the amount of each dosha in our constitution.

Vata, pitta, and kapha make up our unique mind-body type. Every individual has varying amounts of the three doshas. Each one of us has a spectrum of vata, pitta, and kapha that creates our unique and individual qualities. It is the doshas that give us our individual traits and features. Each dosha is associated with particular qualities that manifest in the body and mind. Dryness, for example, is a vata quality. Someone who has vata as their predominant dosha may have more issues related to dryness, such as dry skin or hair or dry, cracking joints. Heat is a pitta quality, so someone who is predominantly pitta may have more issues related to heat. Heaviness is a kapha quality, so someone who is predominantly kapha may feel heavier than a vata or pitta person. We all have unique characteristics that are determined by the amount of vata, pitta, and kapha within our constitution.

Outside the body, doshas connect us to our environment. According to Ayurvedic thought, we are a microcosm within a macrocosm. What exists in the external world exists within each of us. The doshas are affected by the season, time of day, and stage of life. In the fall when it's dry and windy, vata will naturally increase in the body. In the summer when it's warm and the sun is closer, pitta increases. In the spring when it's damp, kapha will increase. In Ayurveda, there are five elements within the universe: earth, water, fire, air, and ether. These elements form everything in nature, as well as within us.

Vata: The Dosha of Movement

The vata dosha contains the elements of air and ether. These are the lightest elements. Therefore, they impart a light, breezy quality to vata. Vata moves like the wind, constantly changing and shifting things around. Just as the wind can cause the environment to become dry, rough, cold, and hard, vata within the body causes dryness, roughness, and coldness.

A person in whom vata dominates will usually be taller or shorter than the average adult, and will typically have been thin as a child. A vata person may have prominent bones and dry joints that crack as they move. They usually have narrow shoulders and hips. Vatas have cool, thin, rough, dry skin and have a tendency to tan or have darker skin, as well as prominent veins. Vatas tend to be cold and suffer from poor circulation in the extremities. They have curly, kinky, coarse, dry hair that's dark brown or black. Their teeth are usually large, crooked, and protruding. Their eyes are small and unsteady. They are very active but exhaust easily with a restless mind, and they experience extreme moods of hope and fear, fulfillment and insecurity. They are erratic and unpredictable, and their faith changes easily. Their short-term memory is good, but they have difficulty recalling the past.

Vatas' dreams are usually full of action, such as running, jumping, and flying, and they may experience intense nightmares. They are light sleepers with interrupted sleep patterns. Vatas are sensitive people with a low tolerance for pain and loud noise. They generally spend money impulsively and do not manage their finances well. They walk a lot, talk a lot, and complain a lot. They are very intuitive, imaginative, and artistic. They are good at writing poems, creating art, or dancing. The vata person has a mind that is very busy like a bee. They are born worriers and worry about anything and everything. Vatas are good at playing the "What if?" game. All this worrying leaves them feeling anxious and nervous. They are often stressed out over things that never end up happening, so they don't enjoy the present moment.

Understanding the Vata Person
Dominant Elements: air and ether

Vata's Responsibilities in the Body:
- Reduces congestion, toxic buildup, and stagnation
- Creates a feeling of lightness and provides energy
- Works as the communication network throughout the body
- Transports nutrients to the microscopic channels throughout the body
- Qualities: dry, light, cold, rough, subtle, mobile

Signs of Aggravation:
- **Dry**: dry skin, hair, eyes, ears, lips, joints, or stools; bloating, gas, and dehydration
- **Light**: restless or ungrounded mind, dizziness, thinness, weight loss
- **Cold**: cold body, poor circulation, constriction/tightness, pain
- **Rough**: broken, cracked skin, varicose veins
- **Subtle**: tremors, twitching, fear, anxiety, insecurity
- **Mobile**: racing mind, restlessness, chattering, fidgeting, obsessive compulsiveness, bipolar disorder, manic depression, muscle twitching, palpitations

Causes of Aggravation:
- Dry, bitter, pungent, astringent, light, cold, stale, or processed foods
- Cold drinks
- Recreational drugs
- Wind, cold, or darkness
- Loud music or bright lights
- Too much screen time (TV, computer, phone, tablet)
- Erratic work/lifestyle schedule

- Fasting and incorrect dieting
- Interrupted or insufficient sleep
- Excessive exercise, running, or staying up late
- Holding back natural urges
- Stress, fear, anxiety, insecurity, or worry
- Overindulgence in sex

Vata is responsible for movement and communication, as it carries messages throughout the body. It controls the downward flow of energy in the pelvis, including elimination, urination, menstruation, and childbirth. When vata increases in the pelvis, it causes frequent urination—a classic symptom of type 2 diabetes.

Vata is the current that carries blood and nervous impulses. When vata becomes disrupted in the nervous system, it can cause numbness in the legs and feet and disturbances in blood flow and digestion. Vata also controls upward and outward actions, such as exhaling, coughing, and speaking. It controls the movement of food through the digestive system and the inhalation of the breath. Vata's airy and mobile qualities can make a person feel anxious and nervous, which can cause them to overeat to help ground themselves. Overindulgence in food is commonly found in type 2 diabetes, indicating a potential vata imbalance. At the cellular level, vata regulates the actions of molecules, nutrients, and waste products. When vata is in balance, we feel creative, energetic, and full of life. But when vata is out of balance, it can cause fatigue, which is a classic symptom of type 2 diabetes.

Pitta: The Dosha of Metabolism

The fire and water elements combine to form the pitta dosha. This dosha is important for the processes of transformation, metabolism, and nutrient assimilation. Pitta controls digestion and biochemical processes in the body. It is the only dosha that contains the fire element. Therefore, pitta is primarily associated with heat.

A person in whom pitta dominates will have a medium build, height, and bone structure. Their skin is generally soft, oily, and warm to the touch, with a reddish or yellowish hue. Pittas have fair complexions and sunburn easily. They often sweat because they have a lot of internal heat. Their hair is also soft and oily—usually reddish or blonde, with a tendency to bald and gray early because they are hot headed. They have moderate-sized, yellowish teeth with soft gums that bleed easily. Sharpness is the main pitta personality trait and physical feature; they have sharp noses, eyes, chins, and unfortunately a sharp tongue as well.

Their eyes are light blue, green, or hazel, with a sharp, penetrating gaze.

Pitta people are good speakers and get straight to the point of the conversation. They have strong, sharp appetites and need large meals to feel satiated, but they do not like to snack. Because of their strong appetite, they become extremely irritable when hungry. They have frequent bowel movements with soft, oily, loose discharges and must evacuate immediately when they feel the urge.

They are moderately active but intensely competitive. They can be overly aggressive or assertive and highly intelligent and organized. They become teachers, doctors, lawyers, and politicians. They can be callous and are easily irritated, and they can even become violent when jealous. They know how to save, but they usually purchase luxuries that make a statement about their position in life to enhance their ego.

The pitta mind is like a bull; once it is set, it is difficult to change. Pitta people are often witty. However, when they are out of balance, they tend to be opinionated, critical, irritable, and quick to anger. They tend to get mad when things don't go their way.

Understanding the Pitta Person
Dominant Elements: fire and water

Pitta's Responsibilities in the Body:
- Maintains acidity of digestive enzymes, breaks down fats, and helps with digestion
- Provides luster to the skin
- Transforms food into energy
- Illuminates intelligence and life
- Provides warmth to the body

Qualities: oily, sharp, hot, light, mobile, liquid, acidic smell

Signs of Aggravation:
- **Oily**: nausea, vomiting, diarrhea, oily skin, skin blisters
- **Sharp**: gastritis, ulcers, acid reflux, heartburn, irritability, anger, sharp pain, sharp headaches
- **Hot**: fevers, infections, inflammations, excessive perspiration, red eyes, desire for cold drinks, thirst, hyperacidity, insomnia
- **Light**: dizziness, sensitivity to heat and light, ringing in the ears
- **Acidic**: acidic smell to sweat and urine, yellow hue to the skin
- **Liquid**: excessive perspiration, thirst, or urination

Causes of Aggravation:

- Summer
- Very sour, salty, or pungent foods, such as yogurt, sour juices, or junk food
- Alcohol, smoking, or excessive drugs
- Outdoor activities in the sun, overexposure to sunlight
- Anger, irritability, intellectual stimulation, competition

The inflammation associated with type 2 diabetes is caused by a pitta imbalance. Decades ago, researchers identified higher levels of inflammation in people with type 2 diabetes. Pitta creates these inflammatory chemicals, which are often higher in people with type 2 diabetes than in people without it.

Pitta's fire is responsible for breaking down and metabolizing food. Pitta is engaged in hormone production, metabolism, and glucose uptake. Insulin is a pitta hormone. Insulin has many roles, but mainly it controls how the body uses carbohydrates. Carbohydrates are in most grains, flours, sugar, and starchy vegetables. The body breaks carbohydrates down into a type of sugar called glucose. Glucose is the primary source of energy used by the body. Insulin acts as a helper for glucose, escorting it into muscle cells for energy. Insulin also brings glucose into the liver, where it is stored and used during times of fatigue. Without insulin, cells are unable to use glucose from carbohydrates. Therefore, if pitta is not functioning correctly, insulin will not be able to do its job, and blood glucose levels will remain high.

The liver is a pitta organ, and it has a special job when it comes to glucose. When blood glucose levels are high, the liver responds to the hormone insulin and absorbs glucose. The liver is like a warehouse for glucose; it releases stored glucose when the body needs it. When the liver is healthy, it can make glucose. Glucose storage is a critical function that keeps people alive when food is scarce. In people with type 2 diabetes, however, pitta may cause dysfunction by causing the liver to abnormally process and produce glucose. This malfunction contributes to blood glucose issues.

Pitta is responsible for the metabolic conversions in the liver and digestive system that the body uses to create energy from carbohydrates. Pitta is also responsible for emotional digestion. Emotional digestion is a process that happens as we digest thoughts and feelings in the mind. Emotional digestion helps us process emotions to bring us to a resolution. Just as the digestive system breaks down and digests food, the mind dissects and digests emotions. When pitta is in balance, it provides power, creates luster in the skin, and maintains body temperature. However, when pitta is out of balance, it can cause inflammation, poor liver functioning, decreased insulin production, and inadequate digestion of carbohydrates.

Kapha: The Dosha of Structure

Kapha, the third dosha, is composed of the water and earth elements. The earth element makes kapha the heaviest of the doshas, and the water element provides dampness and lubrication. Kapha is responsible for growth, structure, and protection. Kapha governs the cerebrospinal fluid, which offers protection for the brain and spinal column. The mucosal lining of the stomach is another protective tissue controlled by kapha.

A person in whom kapha dominates is large, thick, big boned, and strong. Their features are rounded—round face, big eyes, round nose—with an overall sweetness. Kaphas are average height with a tendency to be overweight. They can almost gain weight just by thinking of food!

Their skin is thick, smooth, oily, cool, and usually pale. Their hair is thick and healthy. They seldom get a cavity and have beautiful, even, white teeth. Their eyes are large and well-formed with ample whites and deep blue irises, decorated with thick, long lashes.

Kaphas prefer to remain physically inactive. However, they are healthiest when they exercise and do not overeat. They rarely drink liquids and have one large bowel movement daily. Kapha people in general are slow, steady, and reliable. To understand concepts, they must study repeatedly, but once they comprehend and memorize information, they never forget it. They are extremely compassionate, forgiving, loving, and patient; and they make good nurses, social workers, and clergy members. They have a deep, steady faith and highly developed spiritual feelings.

Kaphas are good with money, but they know how to save to an extreme and can become overly greedy and attached. Their sleep is deep and long, and they dream of romantic settings. They speak slowly in a monotonous voice. Kapha people are loving, nurturing, and caring and play the role of the peacemaker. Kapha personalities like to rely on others and follow others' lead. The kapha mind tends to live in the past. Kapha people get attached and have a hard time letting go.

Understanding the Kapha Person

Dominant Elements: water and earth

Kapha's Responsibilities in the Body:
- Supports the body

- Maintains body lubrication; lubricates the joints
- Develops and strengthens the tissues
- Gives stamina
- Creates forgiveness, love, compassion, calmness, happiness, and contentment

Qualities: moist, cold, heavy, soft, sticky, dull, static, cloudy, slow

Signs of Aggravation:
- **Moist**: clammy skin, mucus
- **Cold:** cold body, coughs, colds, congestion, sinus congestion
- **Heavy**: heaviness, obesity, lethargy, weak digestion, fungal infections (e.g., *Candida albicans*), food allergies
- **Static**: laziness, lethargy
- **Soft**: white-coated tongue, soft frame
- **Liquid**: swelling of the joints, water retention

Causes of Aggravation:
- Rainy weather in late winter and early spring
- Sweet, sour, or salty food; junk food, candy, ice cream, desserts, donuts, fried foods, red meat, milk, and cheese
- Excessive eating and drinking
- Excessive sleep
- Lack of physical activity

Kapha is responsible for growth, stability, structure, cohesion, and protection. The kapha dosha forms and maintains body mass and shape and flexibility in the joints. At the cellular level, kapha engages in the process of converting food into body mass. Most experts consider kapha to be the primary dosha responsible for type 2 diabetes. When there is excess kapha in the body, it contributes to body mass. Kapha governs the physical structure of the body and can manifest in weight gain, lethargy, and resistance to change. Ayurveda identifies many kapha behaviors and foods as factors that may contribute to the development of type 2 diabetes.

When kapha is out of balance, it can affect vata and pitta. Fat is a kapha tissue, but it produces the pitta hormones that contribute to the inflammation associated with type 2 diabetes. As you can see, we need all the doshas to be in balance to maintain healthy physiological functions. If vata, pitta, or kapha is awry, it can create a complicated web of symptoms.

Type 2 diabetes is a complex and multifaceted disorder that is unique to each individual and involves many different body systems and organs. Imbalanced doshas are the underlying energies that cause the body to malfunction. Therefore, it is imperative to address the doshas to correct the imbalance. According to Ayurveda, certain lifestyle behaviors and foods cause the doshas to malfunction and lead to poor health. Through the Ayurvedic lens, we can investigate daily routines and dietary habits to discover the root causes of type 2 diabetes.

The Ayurvedic tradition emphasizes the importance of keeping the three doshas balanced and in harmony. When vata, pitta, or kapha is out of balance, Ayurveda offers specific lifestyle, nutritional, and herbal guidelines to assist the individual in equalizing their constitution. What makes us unique is that we each contain distinct proportions and qualities of the vata, pitta, and kapha doshas.

Your Constitution

Your mind-body type, or constitution, is determined by the unique combination of the doshas present at your conception. Your constitution determines your individuality and is akin to your genetic makeup. Studies have even shown that there is a significant correlation between an individual's constitution and their genes. A person's constitution may include any combination of the doshas, resulting in their unique qualities and defining characteristics.

The ratio of the doshas varies within each person, and Ayurveda acknowledges that these unique combinations make up our diversity. Most individuals have a dual-type constitution and have multiple dominant dosha characteristics. Under certain conditions, one dosha will dominate, and, in other circumstances, the other dosha prevails. The dosha or doshas that are out of balance will determine the type of type 2 diabetes a person is experiencing. Ayurveda aims to rebalance the doshas and bring the person back to their true nature.

Our true constitution is constant, meaning we have the same constitution for our entire life. However, our doshas are in dynamic fluctuation. Age, diet, lifestyle, seasons, and circadian rhythms can all cause the doshas to increase and decrease, resulting in a present state that has deviated from the true nature or constitution we were born with. The optimal functioning of each dosha is essential for good health. Imbalances or disturbances between doshas contribute to many diseases.

When a person is out of balance, their doshas will determine the type and nature of the disease. For example, nervous disorders suggest an imbalance of vata. Inflammation and other conditions associated with heat are caused by an imbalance of pitta. Obesity and disorders related to overindulgence are caused by a kapha imbalance. A specific illness manifests when a particular dosha accumulates or becomes deficient and causes harm to the tissues in the body. In some cases, external factors may trigger the imbalance of the doshas and weaken the body.

Ayurvedic doctors look for clinical signs and symptoms to determine which dosha is out of balance and then make a diagnosis and provide a treatment plan. Two individuals with the same disease may be treated with very different approaches. The constitution, imbalances, and nuances of disease development are specific to each person and merit a personalized treatment plan.

While it is essential to know your constitution, it is equally important, if not more so, to know your current state, including when you are out of balance. Life is a balancing act. The sooner you can detect when you are out of balance, the easier it will be to bring yourself back into balance. Life is dynamic, always changing. That is why it is essential to check in with yourself so that you can bring yourself back into equilibrium. Each meal, each day, provides a new opportunity to either follow your body's natural cues toward well-being or ignore the signs and symptoms and fall further out of balance.

CHAPTER 2

PRAMEHA: THE ORIGINAL TYPE 2 DIABETES

Classic Ayurvedic texts provided detailed recommendations on diet, lifestyle, herbal therapies, and detoxification to prevent and reverse the progression of *prameha*—what we now recognize as type 2 diabetes. Ancient Ayurvedic doctors were able to diagnose type 2 diabetes by observing precise changes in the color, density, and other qualities of patients' urine at a time when computer diagnostics and laboratory tests were not yet available. Ayurvedic doctors relied solely on their sharp senses and intuitive minds to diagnose patients.

Ancient rishis were enlightened Ayurvedic doctors who were tuned into the subtle energy of the doshas. They used their keen sense of awareness to determine the early signs and symptoms of type 2 diabetes. Within nature, we can find many clues that help us understand the inner workings of the human body. Rishis discovered that ants were attracted to the urine of people with type 2 diabetes. In the body's effort to find balance, it expels excess glucose through urine. Ants are attracted to the sweet scent and taste of diabetic urine, and this was used as an indication of excess glucose in patients with type 2 diabetes.

Ancient Ayurvedic physicians were aware of the presence of sugar in blood and urine. They understood that excess glucose was unassimilated by the body and expelled through urine. Today, modern diagnostics such as the urine specific gravity test are used to determine the presence of sugar in the urine and diagnose type 2 diabetes.

The Six Stages of Type 2 Diabetes

Ayurveda truly is preventative medicine. It recognizes the early stages of imbalance long before Western medicine. Symptoms are the body's way of letting us know there is an imbalance. Rather than merely suppressing symptoms, Ayurveda investigates a person's diet and lifestyle to find the root causes of their malady. Ancient Ayurvedic doctors clearly defined a wide variety of symptoms to diagnose a person in the initial stages of type 2 diabetes. By identifying these early signs, they had a better chance of reversing the disease process.

Diet and lifestyle behaviors that contribute to type 2 diabetes include those that increase kapha in the body, such as sweet foods, sedentary habits, and lack of exercise. Kapha naturally embraces damp and heavy qualities, and, according to Ayurvedic theory, "like increases like." Eating heavy foods increases heaviness in the body. Consuming heavy, sweet foods and participating in sedentary activities increase the heavy quality of kapha. Kapha is the dosha that most contributes to type 2 diabetes. Western medicine has also found that sedentary habits and indulgence in sweet, high-glycemic foods promote the development of type 2 diabetes. It recognizes that a high-carbohydrate diet is one of the major causes of the imbalance.

Oversaturation—Too Much of a Not-So-Good Thing

Many diseases prevalent in modern society, such as heart disease, obesity, metabolic syndrome, and type 2 diabetes, can be a result of oversaturation, which means too much of a not-so-good thing. Eating processed and refined foods results in consuming an abundance of empty calories. If the body cannot metabolize and utilize these calories, oversaturation occurs, and waste byproducts develop in the body.

Oversaturation happens when a person overeats, eats foods that are not compatible with their constitution, or eats when they are not hungry. If you have ever gorged and ended up feeling tired and bloated, that was due to oversaturation and the accumulation of metabolic waste. Most sweet, heavy, oily foods can cause a buildup of metabolic waste because they are difficult to digest. Obesity, heaviness, drowsiness, sleepiness, and lethargy are all due to oversaturation and the development of metabolic waste.

In the example of type 2 diabetes, the metabolic waste is excessive blood sugar. The body is not able to properly assimilate and convert all the sugar in the blood into energy. The excess sugar then becomes a waste product that circulates throughout the body, causing damage.

Blood sugar has damp, heavy, sticky, and slimy qualities. When it accumulates in the body, it makes us feel lethargic and tired. It impedes the flow of the doshas and causes blockages, poor circulation, inflammation, and swelling. As metabolic waste accumulates in the stomach, signs of indigestion develop. Digestion becomes stagnant and slow. After meals, you may feel as though you have a heavy rock sitting in your stomach. Elimination can also become slow, and constipation or loose stools with inflammation can develop.

The Ayurvedic perspective on type 2 diabetes considers that body tissues have an optimal level of moisture. Moisture in the stomach promotes digestion when it is within an optimal range. But when metabolic waste accumulates with kapha in the stomach, the combination creates a heavy, damp, sticky substance that extinguishes the digestive fire. A weak digestive fire cannot break down food. This causes more metabolic waste to accumulate, further depleting the strength of digestion. The accumulation of metabolic waste and the strength of digestion are interdependent. Impaired digestion creates a buildup of waste in the body, which depletes the strength of digestion even more. See Figure 2.1. It's this vicious cycle of a low digestive fire and a buildup of toxic waste that initiates the first stage of the disease process.

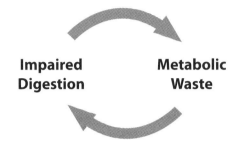

Impaired Digestion   **Metabolic Waste**

Figure 2.1 The Vicious Cycle

Without proper corrections, the digestive fire continues to diminish, and metabolic waste overflows out of the stomach into the pancreas and liver. Metabolic waste damages the tissues of these organs so that they are not able to function properly. The pancreas becomes less efficient at producing insulin. Because of their sticky, slimy, heavy, and cold qualities, waste byproducts create blockages and cause stagnation in the liver, inhibiting detoxification and other natural bodily processes.

If not corrected, metabolic waste and glucose enter the bloodstream and circulate throughout the body, wreaking havoc on weak tissues. At this stage, the imbalance can affect many different body systems, such as the nervous, musculoskeletal, and urinary systems, and cause classic type 2 diabetes symptoms such as blurry vision, dry mouth, numbness in the hands and feet, and frequent urination.

One primary function of the kidneys is to regulate the water content in the body. As glucose enters the bloodstream, the kidneys work diligently to filter it out, resulting in frequent urination. According to Ayurveda, frequent urination is a symptom of the final stage of type 2 diabetes. However, Western medicine considers frequent urination to be an early sign of the disease.

The Six Stages

1. **Accumulation**: Oversaturation of kapha foods and poor lifestyle choices reduce the strength of digestion.
2. **Aggravation**: Metabolic waste forms and kapha increases in the stomach.
3. **Overflowing**: A sticky mass of metabolic waste and kapha overflows from the stomach into the liver and pancreas, affecting detoxification and insulin production.
4. **Spreading**: Glucose enters the bloodstream, causing inflammation throughout the body.
5. **Relocating**: Damage occurs in the weak tissues of the body.
6. **Manifestation**: Classic type 2 diabetes symptoms appear.

To correct type 2 diabetes, Ayurveda removes the root cause and strengthens digestion. The root cause is usually the kapha foods and lifestyle, but Ayurveda also explores a person's sleep habits, stress level, daily routine, and constitution to find out where additional imbalances may lie. Ayurveda uses culinary herbs and spices before meals, mindful eating, and walks after meals to strengthen digestion. Detoxification is an important part of the Ayurvedic program. Detoxification removes blockages caused by waste byproducts and balances the doshas. Once the metabolic waste is removed, the organs can function optimally. The digestive fire is balanced, and carbohydrates and sugar are properly metabolized. Efficient digestion puts an end to the production of metabolic waste, and the cycle is broken.

Why Type 2 Diabetes Is Unique to You

Ayurveda places a strong emphasis on diet and lifestyle as contributing factors for type 2 diabetes. Food can be either medicine or poison, depending on a person's unique constitution and the imbalance(s) they are experiencing. Two people with the same disease can have very different symptoms. Type 2 diabetes can include a large, diverse array of symptoms, involving many different organs and body systems. Ayurvedic theory explains this phenomenon through *khavagunya*, meaning "a weak tissue." The weak tissue in the body can be hereditary or congenital or due to trauma, diet, lifestyle, or stress. We each have a constitution with its strengths and weaknesses. Each person has a propensity toward imbalance depending on genetics, environment, dietary habits, daily routine, and lifestyle choices. A weak tissue can exist in any part of our body or mind. And because there is a weakness, those tissues have a likelihood to develop some type of dysfunction. The dysfunction will vary depending on the doshas involved. But it is the weak tissue that makes certain areas more susceptible to damage from blood sugar.

Blood sugar causes imbalances depending on the location of the weak tissue. Because there is a loss of integrity in that tissue, blood glucose and other waste byproducts will accumulate in that area. Diseases of oversaturation include a buildup of metabolic waste, which causes heaviness in the body and results in a person feeling drowsy and tired. Metabolic waste can also accumulate in the mind. Mental congestion causes brain fog and difficulty concentrating, which are common symptoms of type 2 diabetes.

Ayurveda identifies foods and activities that contribute to the buildup of metabolic waste. This accumulation of biological waste obstructs the downward flow of energy, affecting urination. The kidneys work excessively to filter blood saturated with metabolic waste, so kidney diseases are common in type 2 diabetes. One of the functions of the kidneys is to release a hormone called erythropoietin (EPO), which signals the bone marrow to make more red blood cells. If the kidneys are compromised, they don't send out enough EPO to keep up with physical needs. Anemia is therefore commonly seen in people with type 2 diabetes. It is fascinating that ancient Ayurvedic doctors discovered this connection long before the advent of laboratory procedures.

Types of Diabetes According to Ayurveda

Western medicine recognizes three types of diabetes: type 1, type 2, and gestational. Ayurveda, on the other hand, recognizes three main categories and twenty types of diabetes, depending on the dosha involved:

- Ten kapha-type diabetes
- Six pitta-type diabetes
- Four vata-type diabetes

Kapha-Type Diabetes

Kapha is responsible for structure and cohesiveness in the body, so when diabetes is due to kapha, it affects the integrity of the fat, skin, muscle, and connective tissue, causing those tissues to become lax and loose. Kapha's soft, oily, heavy, static, slow, and smooth qualities promote the growth of diabetic boils and soft, tumorous masses. As fat and liquid merge and intermingle, they cause the muscle tissue to soften and lose integrity, producing laxity within the musculoskeletal system.

As previously mentioned, the examination of urine is a tool used to diagnose diabetes. When kapha enters the urinary system, water and fat combine, creating a substance that causes blockages in the urinary channel. Kapha imparts a cloudy quality to urine, giving it an opaque appearance.

Factors Known to Cause Kapha-Type Diabetes
- Sweet foods
- Obesity
- Sedentary lifestyle
- Emotional eating
- Stress
- High triglycerides

Pitta-Type Diabetes

Because pitta has the fire element and is associated with heat, pitta-type diabetes involves inflammation. When a person's pitta is too high, they are prone to infections and other inflammatory diseases. Inflammation is commonly experienced with type 2 diabetes because the person develops insulin resistance, and their body is not able to efficiently remove sugar from the bloodstream. This causes an inflammatory reaction in the fat cells of the body. Excess body fat, especially abdominal fat, creates a low level of inflammation that interferes with insulin's action and contributes to the disease.

In pitta-type diabetes, inflammation in the nervous system can affect the hands, feet, eyes, and kidneys. Diabetic neuropathy, retinopathy, and nephropathy are painful conditions that affect up to 50 percent of people with type 2 diabetes. Given the complex anatomy of the nervous system, diabetic neuropathy is associated with a wide range of symptoms, but it mostly affects the hands and feet. Diabetic retinopathy affects the eyes. It is a common complication of type 2 diabetes and the leading cause of blindness among the working-age population. Development of diabetic retinopathy and diabetic nephropathy, the leading cause of kidney disease, are both due to the inflammation of pitta.

Factors Known to Cause Pitta-Type Diabetes
- Pancreatic dysfunction
- Stress
- Irregular mealtimes
- Lack of exercise
- Acidic pH

Vata-Type Diabetes

Diet, lifestyle, resisting natural urges, and certain mental tendencies are the root causes of vata-type diabetes. Eating kapha foods and participating in sedentary activities create metabolic waste that causes blockages in the body. These blockages start in the muscle and fat tissues and continue to disrupt the body as they work their way into the nervous system. Vata is the energy responsible for transportation, so when there are blockages in the nervous system, vata is unable to communicate with those areas, which can result in a loss of sensation. Once metabolic waste has made its way to the nervous system, it can cause nerve damage, resulting in a loss of feeling in the feet and legs and making balance unsteady and walking difficult. As these symptoms progress, they may lead to an increased risk of falls.

Factors Known to Cause Vata-Type Diabetes
- Overeating
- Lack of exercise
- Weak digestion
- Anxiety
- Insufficient insulin production
- Resisting the urge to urinate or defecate

Ayurvedic healthcare is patient-centered. It takes a close look at the person's unique constitution, the doshas that created the imbalance(s), the state of the bodily tissues, and the strength of the digestive fire. While there are vata, pitta, and kapha types of diabetes, a person may experience any combination of symptoms and have multiple doshas out of balance.

CHAPTER 3

AYURVEDIC TREATMENTS FOR TYPE 2 DIABETES

Dietary Guidelines

The standard American diet (SAD) is high in artificial ingredients and preservatives, genetically modified organisms, and refined sugars. Within one generation of the introduction of processed foods, many diseases of oversaturation such as type 2 diabetes have quickly spread around the world. The more foods are transformed from their natural state, the less ability they have to nourish the body and the more they become toxic burdens. Processed foods create waste products the body is unable to process, obstructing channels and blocking vital nutrients from reaching minute areas of the body.

Modern eating habits are one of the fundamental causes of the prevalence of type 2 diabetes. According to the classic Ayurvedic texts, "A good and proper diet in disease is worth a hundred medicines, and no amount of medication can do a patient good who does not observe a strict regimen of diet." Ayurveda emphasizes the importance of food as medicine to reverse type 2 diabetes. Herbs are useless without accompanying dietary changes.

According to Ayurveda, people should pay particular attention to the strength of their digestive fire. Start with a light diet and gradually increase the quantity of food. Eating dense foods that are difficult to digest will dampen the digestive fire. The goal is to keep digestion balanced and robust. Since type 2 diabetes is a metabolic disorder, special attention is placed on the state of digestion and assimilation. Eating appropriate quantities, following a regular meal schedule, and sticking to an appropriate diet will help bring the digestive fire into balance.

The Six Tastes

Ayurveda focuses on the six tastes—sweet, sour, salty, pungent, bitter, and astringent—and their effects on the doshas regarding health and wellness. The first three tastes—sweet, sour, and salty—are heavy and increase kapha. The last three—bitter, pungent, and astringent—are light and decrease kapha. The bitter and astringent tastes are most important for alleviating type 2 diabetes because they are light and easy to digest. They reduce kapha and treat the disease by removing excess water. These tastes have a drying action on moisture, fat, muscle, bone marrow, feces, and urine. This helps balance the excess waste, fat, and urine present in type 2 diabetes. Bitter and astringent can easily be digested and assimilated, so they are beneficial for those with impaired digestion.

Recommended Foods for Type 2 Diabetes

- Barley
- Jackfruit
- Bitter melon
- Fenugreek
- Turmeric
- Ginger
- Cinnamon
- Fibrous, bitter green vegetables
- Mung beans
- Poultry

Diet plays a vital role in the prevention and management of type 2 diabetes. The search for foods to treat type 2 diabetes has been a significant focus of scientific research around the world. Improving diet is a traditional, affordable approach used for the management and treatment of type 2 diabetes worldwide. But there is no "one diet fits all" approach to treating this condition. The same food can have various effects on blood glucose depending on a person's constitution and the strength of their digestion.

Western nutrition commonly uses the glycemic index (GI) and glycemic load (GL) of an individual food to determine how it will affect blood sugar. Foods with a low GI and low GL do not raise blood glucose as much as foods with a high GI. Foods with a low GI or GL are generally rich in dietary fiber, which lowers the risk of type 2 diabetes and insulin sensitivity. Whole grains are a significant source of dietary fiber and tend to have low GI values. Ancient whole grains, such as amaranth, barley, and quinoa, have a high fiber content, as well as a low GI and GL. And research has found that regular consumption of specific whole grains decreases the risk of type 2 diabetes by as much as 31 percent.

Barley *(Hordeum vulgare)*

Barley is a highly recommended dietary staple for those with type 2 diabetes. It has a minimal effect on fasting blood glucose, and it can balance blood sugar. Barley is also recommended for obesity and oversaturation, which are two imbalances that commonly coincide with type 2 diabetes. Barley has the highest amount of dietary fiber among the cereals, and it is the world's fourth-most produced cereal crop after wheat, rice, and corn.

Barley is high in antioxidants, making it beneficial for the prevention of type 2 diabetes and metabolic syndrome, as well as other diseases caused by oxidative stress damage such as stroke, Alzheimer's disease, Parkinson's disease, and cancer. Experts attribute this property to saponarin, a flavonoid (plant pigment) with potent antioxidant activity found in barley.

Barley is a rich source of magnesium, a mineral that acts as a co-factor, or helper, for more than 300 enzymes, including those involved in glucose metabolism and insulin secretion. It is also an excellent source of soluble fibers, selenium, phosphorus, and copper—all of which have demonstrated effects on metabolic syndrome, lipid metabolism, and bowel function.

Barley has a wonderfully nutty flavor and a chewy, hearty texture. It comes in two forms: pearl and hulled. Hulled is the more nutritious option—it retains the bran and endosperm layer of the grain. Hulled requires a longer cook time. Polished pearl barley removes the bran layer and has less fiber, so it is therefore less effective in balancing blood sugar. The research used to support the benefits of barley for type 2 diabetes is based on hulled barley. Pearled barely may have some effect, but with the bran layer removed, it will not be as effective. When working to balance blood sugar, use hulled barley.

Cook barley similar to rice. Just bring the water to a boil, add the barley, reduce to a simmer, cook until tender, and serve hot or at room temperature. Alternatively, you can cook it in a slow cooker overnight, so it will be ready in the morning for a quick breakfast or lunch.

HOW TO COOK BARLEY

Ingredients:
- 3 cups water
- 1 cup hulled barley

Instructions: Bring water to a boil in a large saucepan over high heat. Stir in barley, cover, and reduce heat to medium-low. Simmer for 40 to 50 minutes or until tender. The barley will be slightly chewy when done.

Barley is an excellent food to include in your diet. I encourage you to try a variety of recipes with barley for breakfast, lunch, and dinner. Once you find a few recipes you like, keep them in your weekly meal rotation. Include barley in a variety of ways:
- Breakfast grain
- Soups and stews

- Replacement for rice and other grains
- Bread, biscuits, and muffins made with barley
- Salads
- With soft-boiled, scrambled, or poached eggs
- Polenta-style barley cakes

Barley bread can be a powerful, blood-sugar-balancing tool. Eating bread containing barley improves metabolism and decreases blood sugar. It also feeds beneficial gut bacteria that work to curb cravings. Research indicates that eating bread made from barley kernels at breakfast, lunch, and dinner can reduce blood sugar and insulin levels, increase insulin sensitivity, and suppress the appetite for up to 14 hours. Eating barley bread also increases hormones in the gut that regulate metabolism and appetite and reduce inflammation. Swedish researchers discovered that dietary fibers from barley increase *Prevotella copri,* a beneficial bacterium in the gut that regulates blood sugar and decreases harmful gut bacteria. Interested in trying barley bread to balance blood sugar? Visit this website (https://cup.org/35jGtDe) for a recipe from the *British Journal of Nutrition.*

Jackfruit *(Articarpus heterophyllus Lam.)*

Jackfruit is an integral part of the standard Indian diet and is available in many health-food stores around the world. It grows in tropical climates and is a rich source of carbohydrates, minerals, dietary fiber, and vitamins.

Jackfruit possesses a wide variety of medicinal properties, such as antibacterial, anti-inflammatory, anti-diabetic, and antioxidant actions. Ayurveda highly recommends jackfruit as a treatment for type 2 diabetes, and studies have confirmed its ability to promote weight loss, improve insulin sensitivity, reduce fat, and manage complications related to type 2 diabetes.

Ayurveda practitioners have used jackfruit tea to treat type 2 diabetes successfully. Jackfruit reduces blood sugar and fat cells. It prevents and manages the symptoms of type 2 diabetes by regulating the release of glucose and insulin in the body to improve insulin sensitivity.

If you live in the tropics, you may be able to find fresh jackfruit. If not, you can buy canned or frozen jackfruit at most health-food stores and online. The ripe fruit tastes sweet and is great alone or blended with other fruits into smoothies. Unripe jackfruit tastes like a mix between shredded chicken and pork. It is an excellent meat substitute for people who don't eat meat. Because it has a neutral flavor and a meat-like texture, unripe jackfruit blends well into dishes and absorbs the flavors of various sauces and condiments. You can mix it into barley soups and stews. Try unripe cooked jackfruit with pesto over spiraled zucchini. There are endless options for creating fun, new meals with jackfruit!

Bitter Melon *(Momordica charantia)*

Bitter melon is a tendril-bearing perennial vine that can grow up to 15 feet. It bears elongated fruits with a knobby surface. The fruit has a distinctive bitter taste, which is more pronounced as it ripens, hence the name bitter melon or bitter gourd.

Bitter melon is known for its anti-diabetic properties. Ancient rishis found its bitter taste to be responsible for kindling the digestive fire and reducing kapha and pitta. Abundant clinical studies have shown that the anti-diabetic and hypoglycemic (blood sugar lowering) properties of bitter melon help regenerate the pancreas and reduce insulin resistance. Bitter melon regulates the amount of glucose absorbed by the gut and works in much the same way as insulin to regulate glucose metabolism.

Bitter melon is rich in minerals such as potassium, calcium, zinc, magnesium, phosphorus, and iron. It also contains high amounts of the vitamins C, A, and E, as well as many B vitamins. Bitter melon is an excellent source of dietary fiber and contains a powerful combination of antioxidants, which contribute to its medicinal value.

Modern scientific evidence supports the traditional Ayurvedic uses of bitter melon. More than a hundred research studies worldwide have demonstrated its anti-hyperglycemic and hypoglycemic effects. It inhibits glucose uptake in the intestines, balances fat, reduces the formation of glucose, and preserves the pancreas. It is one of the most promising plants for treating type 2 diabetes. There are more than a thousand herbal products produced worldwide for the treatment of hyperglycemia (high blood sugar), and bitter melon is a prevalent and well-researched resource among them.

Fenugreek *(Trigonella foenum-graecum)*

Fenugreek is an annual herbaceous shrub with small, pale-yellow flowers. Its seeds are a staple for traditional herbal medicine in many cultures. Fenugreek is a digestion-enhancing culinary spice with anti-inflammatory, antioxidant, anti-cancer, and anti-diabetic properties.

Fenugreek can help prevent type 2 diabetes. One to two teaspoons of fenugreek daily can decrease fasting blood glucose, postprandial (post-meal) blood glucose, and LDL cholesterol, reducing the chance of developing type 2 diabetes with no adverse effects.

When using fenugreek seeds, choose whole, unadulterated seeds over degummed seeds. Whole, raw fenugreek seeds, seed powder, and cooked seeds have all been shown to decrease postprandial glucose levels. In contrast, degummed seeds have little influence on glucose. The use of fenugreek for type 2 diabetes is supported by substantial clinical evidence and is practical, affordable, and safe.

Turmeric *(Curcuma longa)*

For thousands of years, Ayurvedic medicine has used turmeric as a treatment for type 2 diabetes. Turmeric is the most widely researched herb in the scientific world. Curcumin, one active plant chemical found in turmeric, has caught scientific attention for its powerful therapeutic effects on blood sugar and cholesterol.

Curcumin balances blood glucose through its ability to regulate the hormones produced by fat tissue. Fat tissue plays an essential role in controlling blood sugar within the entire body by secreting a hormone called adiponectin, which stimulates glucose utilization in the skeletal muscles and the liver, thereby reducing blood glucose.

Curcumin helps manage type 2 diabetes by improving insulin resistance, hyperglycemia, hyperlipidemia (high cholesterol), and pancreas health. Turmeric provides a broad spectrum of benefits in preventing type 2 diabetes and its potential complications.

Ginger *(Zingiber officinale)*

Ginger is a leading ingredient in many Ayurvedic formulas and culinary spices. It is available fresh or as a powder; the powder is spicier. Most research supporting the use of ginger for type 2 diabetes has used ginger powder in the diet to manage postprandial hyperglycemia, blood glucose, insulin sensitivity, and lipid profile.

Researchers credit the beneficial effects of ginger to two compounds: gingerols and shogaol. Of the two, gingerols appear to be the more effective at improving insulin sensitivity. Increasing insulin sensitivity allows the cells of the body to use blood glucose more effectively, which reduces blood sugar. These compounds inhibit carbohydrate metabolism and increase insulin release, resulting in enhanced glucose uptake in fat and muscle tissues. Ginger also has a lipid-lowering effect that improves insulin resistance.

A little bit of ginger goes a long way—just 1 tablespoon of ginger daily can reduce fasting blood glucose, insulin resistance, unhealthy fats such as triglycerides, total cholesterol, and inflammatory markers. Many studies have demonstrated the safety of ginger as a regular dietary addition. To get ginger in your diet, try using it as a culinary spice or make ginger tea. Ginger tastes fantastic and has many benefits for those with type 2 diabetes.

Ginger and cinnamon make a potent combination. They both contain powerful antioxidants that reduce oxidative stress related to type 2 diabetes. When combined, ginger and cinnamon act synergistically and increase the availability of antioxidants compared to using ginger or cinnamon alone. Ginger and cinnamon also support the male reproductive system and increase sperm count in men with type 2 diabetes.

Cinnamon *(Cinnamomum cassia)*

There are about 250 species in the cinnamon family, ranging from shrubs to small- to medium-sized trees. Cinnamon grows in various altitudes and soils throughout tropical rain forests. *Cinnamomum cassia* is a widely researched species with potent blood-glucose-lowering and fat-reducing effects.

Ayurveda uses cinnamon in more than 600 herbal formulations, as it helps with the absorption of complex herbal formulas. It is beneficial for colds and flus, sinus congestion, bronchitis, kidney conditions, hypertension, menstrual cramps, immune function, dental care, and type 2 diabetes. Cinnamon stokes the digestive fire and dispels metabolic waste. It has positive effects on the cardiovascular system and circulation. Cinnamon is a universal medicine, good for the elderly and those with a weak constitution. It has potent anti-microbial, antifungal, antiviral, antioxidant, antitumor, blood-pressure-reducing, cholesterol- and lipid-lowering, hypoglycemic, and gastro-protective properties.

Cinnamon has many benefits when it comes to type 2 diabetes. Similar to ginger, eating cinnamon decreases levels of fasting blood glucose, total cholesterol, and unhealthy fats. Cinnamon promotes insulin-signaling pathways in muscles, enhancing glucose uptake and increasing insulin production.

Some of the beneficial effects of cinnamon on balancing blood sugar levels are due to its polyphenol compounds. These compounds work in several ways. Polyphenol compounds have a powerful antioxidant effect that reduces oxidative stress and inflammation related to type 2 diabetes. These compounds also activate insulin receptors and insulin signaling in the intestinal tract, thereby increasing glucose uptake and reducing post-digestive blood glucose and lipid metabolism.

Just one-quarter teaspoon of cinnamon daily can reduce serum glucose, triglycerides, LDL cholesterol, and total cholesterol in people with type 2 diabetes. It is therefore very beneficial for people who have risk factors associated with cardiovascular disease to include cinnamon in their diet. Metabolic syndrome is associated with insulin resistance, high cholesterol, inflammation, decreased antioxidant activity, and increased weight gain. Taking one-quarter teaspoon of cinnamon daily improves all these conditions. Cinnamon works effectively as a tea or culinary spice.

Fibrous, Bitter, Green Vegetables

Bitter greens gently purify the body. They have a diuretic action that helps remove excess water and metabolic waste from the body, assisting with weight loss. Bitter greens contain vitamins A, C, and K and minerals such as calcium, potassium, and magnesium. In addition to being vitamin-rich, bitter greens are exceptional for digestion. Eating bitter foods stimulates enzyme production and bile flow, promoting healthy digestion. The high fiber content in bitter greens also helps to eliminate waste through the digestive tract.

High-fiber bitter greens induce satiety (the feeling of fullness) because they take a long time to digest. Fiber, in turn, ensures that the greens do not metabolize quickly and do not cause a spike in blood sugar. Bitter greens also have very low glycemic values. Here are some examples of bitter greens to include in your diet:

- Arugula
- Asparagus
- Endive
- Broccoli
- Collard greens
- Dandelion greens
- Green beans
- Escarole
- Kale
- Mustard greens
- Nettles
- Parsley
- Spinach
- Turnip greens
- Watercress

Mung Beans (Mudga)

Mung beans are a staple in the Ayurvedic diet for balancing blood sugar. They possess several properties that help keep blood sugar levels low. Mung beans are high in fiber, with more than 15 grams per cup, which helps reduce blood glucose and triglycerides. Mung beans also contain antioxidants, which lower blood sugar and help insulin work more effectively. They can also reduce plasma C-peptide, an indicator of insulin release, thereby producing measurable improvements in glucose metabolism and insulin sensitivity.

Including mung beans in a diet with high-carbohydrate foods, such as grains, bread, pasta, and breakfast cereals, can lower glucose response by 45 percent and overall postprandial glucose levels in individuals with type 2 diabetes. Eating mung beans regularly is a great way to reduce your overall blood glucose.

The prevalence of type 2 diabetes continues to climb, and pharmaceutical drugs are still the primary form of treatment. But with pharmaceutical interventions come side effects, cost and accessibility issues, and limited effects. Identifying natural, affordable options to treat people worldwide effectively is essential in working with type 2 diabetes. Incorporating dietary interventions into a personalized treatment plan is an integrated and effective approach.

Foods to Avoid

Ayurveda provides guidance on foods to include in the diet, as well as those to avoid. People with type 2 diabetes should avoid eating sweet, heavy, and cooling foods because they dampen the digestive fire. Habitually consuming these foods causes the body to accumulate excess phlegm, bile, and fat. These accumulations interfere with the body's natural rhythms, circulation, and metabolism, leading to glycosuria (the excretion of glucose into the urine).

Ancient Ayurvedic doctors were well aware of the properties of specific foods and the effects they have on blood glucose. They also demonstrated a vast understanding of the physiological processes that occur when consuming these foods. Heavy and cooling foods are challenging to digest. People with type 2 diabetes suffer from a metabolic disturbance. They have difficulty breaking down hard-to-digest foods. If meals are inadequately processed and eliminated from the body, waste starts to accumulate, causing congestion. Blockages in the body interfere with the body's natural functions. When obstructed, energetic pathways get redirected, causing changes in the flow of urine, numbness or loss of sensation in the body, dry skin, or nervous system and cardiovascular disorders.

Foods to Avoid for Type 2 Diabetes:

- Fatty, greasy foods
- Sugar
- Heavy foods
- Pork
- Beef
- Cheese
- Duck
- Milk and milk preparations
- Certain grains and cereals (e.g., white rice, white flour)
- Wine
- Beer
- Molasses

The first step to correcting an imbalance is removing the root cause. These foods are indicated as the root causes of type 2 diabetes, so it is therefore important to eliminate them from the diet. People with type 2 diabetes have a metabolic disorder caused by a weak digestive fire, so their digestion is compromised. All of the contraindicated foods are sweet, cooling, or heavy and thus difficult for someone with type 2 diabetes to digest.

Upgrade Your Lifestyle

By making a few simple lifestyle changes, we could prevent 80 to 90 percent of all cases of type 2 diabetes. A regular exercise program can reduce the need for prescription medications. New evidence suggests that most people with recently diagnosed type 2 diabetes can expect the condition to go into remission after weight reduction and exercise, reducing the need for medication.

People with prediabetes who use weight loss and exercise interventions can reduce the need for metformin (Glucophage) by 80 percent. Even the American Diabetes Association and the European Association for the Study of Diabetes have stated that some patients newly diagnosed with type 2 diabetes "should be given the opportunity to engage in lifestyle changes for 3 to 6 months before embarking on pharmacotherapy." (Nathan 193) These findings are crucial and inspiring! We need to choose healthy meals and engage in daily physical activity to prevent and reverse type 2 diabetes. Modern research is now confirming what Ayurveda found thousands of years ago.

Ayurveda recommends specific exercises for type 2 diabetes that promote the proper utilization of fat and glucose in the body. In the advanced stages of the disease, Ayurveda suggests exercises such as wrestling; playing games; riding an elephant, horse, or cart; digging a well; and walking. People with type 2 diabetes were advised to walk 100 miles barefoot and not stay in one place for more than one night. They were told to live like a sage and only eat foods given to them.

Today, it would be difficult to fully comply with this recommendation. However, the overall message is valid as it encourages people to participate in resistance training and cardiovascular exercise, do daily chores, walk more, and eat a simple diet. Resistance training builds muscle and promotes glycemic uptake. Playing sports and games offers cardiovascular benefits. Doing household chores reduces sedentary behavior. Rather than dig a well, there are many daily chores and activities you can do to burn calories. Daily walking is an easy way to transform your lifestyle into one that helps you overcome type 2 diabetes.

Make Major Strides with Walking

Walking is the most popular physical activity among Americans and is especially beneficial for those with type 2 diabetes. Many experts highly recommend walking because it is a low-impact cardio activity that requires little equipment or training. Walking is an inexpensive, a convenient, and a sustainable form of exercise, bringing many health benefits to people with type 2 diabetes. It lowers pro-inflammatory markers, reduces cardiovascular impairments, decreases cardiovascular mortality, and reduces body mass index (BMI).

Walking for just 2 to 4 hours per week can reduce the risk of developing type 2 diabetes, heart disease, obesity, and metabolic syndrome by 50 percent. Thirty to forty-five minutes of walking three or four times per week can be instrumental in reducing blood glucose levels.

People who are overweight may experience many challenges when it comes to finding a form of exercise that is both enjoyable and beneficial. Walking is ideal because it is a low-impact activity and typically doesn't place excessive stress on the joints. Walking is suitable for aging adults, people prone to joint pain, and anyone hoping to transition from a sedentary lifestyle to a more active one. Walking works large muscle groups such as the quadriceps, hamstrings, and gluteus muscles ("glutes"), which improves glucose uptake, increases circulation, promotes endurance, and reduces obesity and the risk of type 2 diabetes.

Walking can be either a modest form of exercise or a high-intensity activity. The average person burns about 180 calories per half hour of walking. If you walk 10 minutes after breakfast, lunch, and dinner, you could burn 1,260 calories in a week. Dr. Steven Blair at the Institute for Aerobics Research discovered that people who walk 30 minutes per day, 6 days a week, gain the most benefits conferred by exercise. He found that people who engage in this modest amount of activity have the same mortality rate as those who run 30 to 40 miles a week.

Transitioning into a healthy lifestyle is as simple as stepping into it. Most people, regardless of weight, age, gender, or preexisting conditions, can enjoy walking as an activity.

How Constitution Affects the Benefits of Walking

Walking has specific and distinct effects on the body depending on a person's constitution. The Ayurvedic prevention program for individuals at risk for developing type 2 diabetes provides an individualized wellness plan based on the person's unique constitution and current state. Some people may require longer, more intense walks, while others can benefit more from shorter, more frequent walks.

Constitution plays an essential role in metabolic processes, and a person's constitution will determine the effects walking has on blood glucose. People with a vata-pitta constitution have the most significant changes in post-meal blood glucose after walking, indicating that these individuals can easily control blood glucose. Some researchers believe that the action of glucose uptake is due to vata's dynamic movements, which promote the quick utilization of glucose by the skeletal muscles. Vata-pitta people can therefore benefit from a shorter post-meal walking program. People with a kapha constitution may benefit from more extended, strenuous post-meal walking to help move kapha's slow nature and encourage glucose uptake.

A reduction in daily walking is one of the most significant contributing lifestyle factors to the type 2 diabetes epidemic. Since the introduction of powered machinery, daily step numbers have declined by 50 to 70 percent. Many occupations have transitioned from physical labor to sedentary desk work. This reduction in physical activity has a significant impact on health and well-being.

After only a 2-week reduction in physical activity that engages the large muscles, muscle mass begins to deteriorate and fat accumulates. When there is muscle loss, glucose uptake declines, resulting in high blood glucose levels. Reducing daily steps for just 3 weeks increases plasma insulin by 30 percent. Significant physiological changes start after just a couple of weeks, so think of what may happen after 1 or 2 months or even years! Reducing daily steps has considerable health consequences on blood glucose, muscle loss, and body composition, all within a brief period.

With each step you take throughout the day, you travel farther down the path to a healthier lifestyle. Researchers have found that walking about 10,000 steps throughout the day, including both official walks and walking done as part of an active lifestyle, is an effective way to keep blood glucose levels within a healthy range, lower BMI, reduce belly fat, and improve insulin sensitivity. Wearing a pedometer (a device that counts your steps) will help you keep track of your daily steps and stay motivated to keep moving.

An active lifestyle has a positive effect on insulin sensitivity, which is a big problem for pre-diabetic people. Simple ways to include walking in your daily routine include walking while on the phone at work, taking the stairs instead of the elevator, going for a walk after meals, walking your dog, or walking over to a coworker rather than sending an email.

Taking short walks after meals is a proven Ayurvedic practice to promote healthy digestion and prevent type 2 diabetes. The muscle contractions connected with short walks immediately help reduce potentially dangerous levels of post-meal blood glucose. Walking after meals is more effective at lowering blood glucose spikes than pre-meal walking. Walks after heavy, carbohydrate-loaded meals provide the most significant benefits for glucose control. However, it's important to walk after every meal. Research indicates that walking 10 minutes after every meal leads to better blood sugar results than taking one 30-minute walk per day. Walking after meals also improves the process of digestion. Food moves through the digestive system more quickly when you take a short walk after a meal; this can help alleviate feelings of indigestion, stagnation, and oversaturation. Walking after meals is a fantastic habit to get into when transitioning into a healthier lifestyle. Post-meal walks are a crucial part of the blood-sugar-balancing program and are recommended for every constitution. Keep after-meal walks moderate, not strenuous. Too much strenuous activity directly after a meal can impede digestion.

Proven Workouts for Type 2 Diabetes

Physical activity is critical for blood-glucose management and the overall health of people who have prediabetes or type 2 diabetes. Exercise reduces cardiovascular risk factors, promotes weight loss, improves well-being, strengthens the mind-body connection, and helps prevent the development of type 2 diabetes.

Type 2 diabetes is a complex condition with progressive complications that can affect the quality and duration of life. As previously discussed, walking is a beneficial form of exercise for people with type 2 diabetes. Ayurveda also recommends resistance training and cardio workouts for managing this condition.

Resistance training causes muscles to contract against an external opposition and helps increase strength, tone, mass, and endurance. Increased muscle mass results in increased glucose uptake, so exercise programs that build muscle also balance blood glucose.

Resistance training improves strength, reduces injuries, and improves the quality of life in people with type 2 diabetes. It is a quick and effective method to achieve copious health benefits. In just one month, you can reduce complications from type 2 diabetes with resistance training. You can experience improved gait, balance, and muscle strength. Resistance training can improve muscle functioning, thus preventing functional decline and type 2 diabetes complications. Try resistance training at least twice weekly, and be sure to include exercises for all large muscle groups. A combination of resistance training and walking is a very effective way to promote overall physical fitness.

To get the most benefit from your exercise routine, include cardio exercise along with walking and resistance training. This approach provides the most significant reduction in blood sugar levels. Cardio workouts increase blood circulation, and weight training increases strength and muscle tone and stimulates the production of human growth hormones. This combination results in improved posture and protection against injuries that can occur due to loss of muscle tone and bone density.

Diabetes-intervention programs including changes in diet, lifestyle, and exercise reduce the incidence of type 2 diabetes by 58 percent in overweight, glucose-intolerant individuals at high risk for developing diabetes. These programs include a minimum of 150 minutes per week of physical activity, as well as a weight-loss program. Experts recommend that the intensity of the workout starts between 40 and 50 percent of your maximum heart rate and progresses to 70 to 80 percent.

Formulating Your Exercise Program

The American Diabetes Association and most type 2 diabetes experts have repeatedly recommended 120 to 150 minutes of weekly exercise. However, there is no one-size-fits-all exercise program for type 2 diabetes. For maximum benefits, an exercise program should be unique to the individual. The appropriate duration and type of exercise will depend on the person's constitution. Kapha people will experience more significant effects on glycemic control if they exercise 150 minutes per week. Due to their slower metabolism, kapha people need a slightly longer exercise program than vata and pitta people. That extra thirty minutes of weekly exercise can substantially reduce average glucose levels.

Regular physical activity supports immune and hormone function and keeps the body and mind healthy. Exercise plays a significant role in maintaining fitness and balancing weight. A combination of walking and both weight-bearing and cardio exercises will balance blood sugar, increase energy, improve muscle tone and strength, protect against bone density loss, and improve your sense of well-being due to increased endorphin production. Good examples of cardio workouts include hiking, swimming, dancing, aerobics, cycling, and basketball. We all have a unique body type and personality, so some types of cardio workouts may appeal more than others. It's important to find a form of cardio exercise that you enjoy.

Doing any physical activity is better than doing none. The typical modern lifestyle is exceptionally sedentary, and movement is crucial to building muscle, which helps control type 2 diabetes. If you are unsure how much exercise you get, I recommend keeping an exercise journal to monitor your activity. You may be surprised at how little you move in a day.

There are many different activities you can do to reduce sedentary time. The following activities and domestic chores will burn the same amount of calories:

- 30 minutes of dancing
- 20 minutes of tennis
- 17 minutes of uphill hiking
- 15 minutes of swimming
- 40 minutes of housekeeping
- 30 minutes of weeding the garden
- 25 minutes of mowing the lawn
- 15 minutes of shoveling snow

Other ways of fitting physical activity into your day include making the bed, walking instead of driving, carrying groceries home, washing the car at home, and cleaning the garage. It all adds up to movement, which reduces blood glucose.

Every time you climb a set of stairs, you burn more calories than you would by taking the elevator. Walking up stairs provides cardiovascular exercise, increasing the heart rate by 10 beats for every flight climbed. When you engage your calves, thighs, and glutes, they become stronger and more efficient at glucose uptake. Exercise is not just about burning calories; it's also about working muscle groups to retain muscle mass and build new muscle.

Exercise also helps the body detoxify. It enhances the transportation of oxygen and nutrients into cells and transports carbon dioxide and waste products out of the tissues, into the bloodstream, and to the organs of elimination. It also stimulates digestion and bowel movements to prevent toxic buildup.

Regular exercise is an important component of the Ayurveda solution to type 2 diabetes. When weight loss occurs without activity, it is likely due to a loss of lean muscle, not body fat. Body fat stores toxins that cause disease, so burning fat is the primary objective in detoxification, and burning fat requires physical activity. When exercise is part of a weight loss program, body composition improves. There is an increase in lean body mass and a decrease in body fat. Muscle is responsible for the majority of glucose uptake, so more muscle means better glucose uptake and lower blood glucose.

It is better to get a little exercise each day through regular movement than to try to fit it all into one trip to the gym or a fitness class each week. The body responds better to light daily exercise than to spurts of activity followed by periods of sedentary behavior.

Resistance bands are ideal for home exercising. They are fun and provide a good workout for a low cost. Resistance bands are great if you don't have room for a lot of gym equipment. You can use them to do pull-up exercises for the upper body and squats and lunges for the lower body. They easily attach to doorways and can be stored in a closet or drawer when not in use.

Light hand and ankle weights can be used for upper- and lower-body workouts with surprising results. You can use them to do some simple leg lifts and arm movements.

Jumping or bouncing on a rebounder, a type of mini trampoline, is a fun, indoor way to burn calories and stimulate blood circulation. It gets your heart pumping and your lungs working harder. The bouncing movement also stimulates the flow of lymphatic fluids throughout your body, removing toxins and improving immune system function.

There are many online sources for beginner yoga, dance, and other simple fitness routines that are fun and can be completed in 30 minutes or less. You can follow a simple exercise-ball routine and then use it as a chair throughout the day. Exercise balls improve posture and balance and strengthen abdominal muscles.

Stoking Your Brain

Exercise is not only crucial to physical fitness, but also to brain fitness. Our brains require large amounts of oxygen, blood, hormones, and other chemicals to function effectively. Being sedentary not only affects blood glucose but brain functioning as well. A lack of exercise causes us to feel mentally sluggish and less alert. Ayurveda considers "lassitude" to be a root cause of type 2 diabetes. Physical exercise helps your arteries stay clear and clean, so your brain can benefit from an ample delivery of oxygen, nutrients, and hormones. Increased blood circulation to the brain improves metabolism, allowing the brain to work faster and more efficiently. A regular exercise program can stoke your mental fire and reduce lassitude.

Regular exercise keeps your brain "fit" and operating optimally. Exercise exerts its effects on the brain by several mechanisms. It promotes neurogenesis, the growth of new brain cells. Exercise also releases neurotransmitters in the brain that improve memory and cognition and help to reduce physical and mental pain. Endorphin production increases during exercise, which puts us in a positive mood and helps us manage stress better. Increased participation in sports and other physical activities is strongly associated with decreased symptoms of anxiety, depression, lassitude, and insomnia. Those who exercise also have better self-esteem and self-worth, as exercise stimulates mood-enhancing brain chemistry.

Exercise benefits blood glucose and reduces the risks associated with type 2 diabetes. But if a person with type 2 diabetes is not willing to exercise, they will never experience those health benefits. Lassitude can make you feel unmotivated and stop you from participating in physical activity.

Motivational strategies such as the use of coaches, peer support, and step counters are excellent ways to stay on top of your exercise regime. Studies indicate that they are an essential part of lifestyle training for patients with type 2 diabetes. Motivational strategies such as these have been proven effective in increasing daily movement and helping people stick to their exercise program. Qualified coaches for patients with type 2 diabetes can help ensure optimal glycemic control and minimize the risk of injury when starting a new exercise program.

Supervised exercise training helps reduce blood glucose levels and other modifiable cardiovascular risk factors related to type 2 diabetes. Along with counseling, it significantly improves both physical and mental quality of life for those with type 2 diabetes. These motivational strategies can promote permanent lifestyle changes and improve mental health. When starting your exercise program, I highly recommend investing in a personal trainer to help you stay motivated, engaged, and on the right track. It's also good to have an accountability buddy to keep you on top of your workout and walk schedule.

Get Off the Couch

Excessive sedentary behavior increases the risk of developing type 2 diabetes and metabolic syndrome. Ayurveda considers sedentary behaviors such as "sitting on cushions for long periods" to be a contributing factor for type 2 diabetes. Think of the endless number of hours spent on the couch. Excessive time spent watching television, playing video games, and using the computer is a public health issue. Children in the United States spend more time watching TV than on any other activity besides sleep. In some cases, time spent watching television exceeds time spent in school. As the number of hours spent watching television increase, so do blood glucose levels.

People with type 2 diabetes tend to have more sedentary time than people with a healthy glucose metabolism. An extra hour of sedentary time per day has been associated with a 22 percent increased risk of developing type 2 diabetes and a 39 percent increased risk of developing metabolic syndrome. These findings are independent of high-intensity physical activity, which highlights the importance of holistic and complete lifestyle changes. A person with a regular, high-intensity workout is still at risk of developing type 2 diabetes if most of their time spent throughout the day is sedentary.

Understanding the relationship between sedentary behavior and type 2 diabetes can help you prevent or control this disease. It is essential to determine when and where sedentary behaviors occur throughout your day. One thing to think about is sedentary behavior at work. You can reduce sitting in the workplace by trying sit-stand workstations, along with other lifestyle changes that reduce sedentary behavior.

By understanding more about our bodily processes, we can better understand the relationship between sedentary behavior and type 2 diabetes. The activity—or inactivity—of muscle cells plays an essential role in glucose metabolism. Insulin stimulates muscles to take up glucose, and the muscular system is responsible for the uptake of 80 to 90 percent of glucose consumed in the diet. Movement is therefore necessary for glucose uptake; if there is no physical movement, blood glucose levels stay elevated and damage occurs. If a person is sedentary after a large meal, the muscular system does not have the opportunity to utilize blood glucose—another reason to take a walk after meals.

The hazardous effects of a sedentary lifestyle on blood glucose exist regardless of high-intensity physical activity. It is therefore crucial to reduce sedentary behavior. Occasionally working out is not enough.

Quality Sleep: Not Just a Dream

According to Ayurvedic theory, sleep is one of the three main pillars of life, and, if "properly indulged, it will support the body, just like a house is supported by its pillars." (Trikamji 358) The doshas regulate moods, mental disposition, brain functioning, and sleep patterns. When the doshas are in balance, we experience good mental and physical health. But when the doshas are out of balance, it can result in changes to various life functions, including sleep.

Ayurveda has many strategies for optimizing the quality of sleep, especially when it comes to balancing the doshas. Each dosha has specific attributes that affect sleep. Vata people have more movement and are more likely to suffer from insomnia and sleep-maintenance issues. According to the *Charaka Samhita*, an ancient Ayurvedic text, vata-dominant people of all ages have poor-quality sleep and often complain of insomnia. Ayurvedic research suggests that the dominance of the vata dosha is a causative factor for insomnia.

But people of all constitutions can have difficulty sleeping. The pitta dosha is associated with heat, and pitta people tend to sleep moderately but are disturbed by their dreams. Pitta people tend to hold their emotions in, so they do a lot of processing of thoughts and interactions in their dreams.

Kapha people tend to have a calm, relaxed temperament and can fall asleep quickly and have better sleep duration with fewer maintenance issues. But kapha people feel heaviness in their mind and body, so they find it challenging to wake. Kapha-dominant individuals will feel more sluggish and unmotivated as the kapha dosha increases. Sleep habits such as napping and excessive sleep intensify the heavy quality of kapha and are causative factors for type 2 diabetes. It's important for kapha people to avoid the urge to oversleep and nap.

Ayurveda offers specific guidelines about the number of hours people should sleep to maintain balance within their constitution. A person with excess kapha will benefit from less sleep than a person with excess vata or pitta. Kapha people should go to bed early and wake before sunrise, sleeping 6 or 7 hours nightly.

Ayurveda texts teach that happiness and unhappiness, proper nourishment or emaciation, strength and debility, sexual powers and impotence, knowledge and ignorance, life and its absence (death)—all are dependent on sleep. This statement provides insight into the overwhelming impact sleep has on life. Rishis believed that sleep provides medicinal value when used properly but can cause harm or even death when misused. Many variables relating to sleep, such as time of day and duration of sleep as well as an individual's age, constitution, and specific imbalance, all have an effect.

Ayurveda provides complete details about who can sleep during the day and who should not. Napping can be beneficial for children, elderly people, and people with wasting diseases or in convalescence. However, people suffering from type 2 diabetes, obesity, conditions of overindulgence, and kapha-related imbalances should not sleep during the day or excessively at night. Daytime napping is a frequent habit among people with type 2 diabetes. Napping, as well as overly short and long periods of sleep, increases the likelihood of developing type 2 diabetes. Napping during the day and sleeping 5 hours or less at night creates the highest risk. The healthiest sleep pattern is 6 or 7 hours of sleep at night, without napping.

The health consequences of sleep habits and how they relate to type 2 diabetes is also a concern known to Western medicine. Many studies have demonstrated an increased risk of type 2 diabetes in those who habitually nap, regardless of cultural norms. Unhealthy sleep habits contribute to metabolic dysfunction, type 2 diabetes, and obesity, regardless of factors such as BMI, diet, and physical activity. In most cases, napping is established years before the onset of type 2 diabetes and has been found to increase the risk of developing type 2 diabetes by as much as 30 percent.

Daytime napping has a direct effect on blood sugar, causing significant rises in blood glucose and insulin levels. The duration of daytime napping also has a profound effect. Napping for longer than 30 minutes increases the risk of abnormal glucose metabolism even more.

Napping and excessive sleep have many effects on the body that can cause a person to become insulin resistant. These improper sleep habits elevate inflammation and raise cortisol, a stress hormone. Waking from a nap causes stress and activates a fight-or-flight response, altering insulin secretion and glycemic control.

Hormonal influences based on circadian rhythms are also responsible for the correlation between daytime napping and type 2 diabetes. The processes involved in sleep have profound impacts on multiple bodily functions, including the release of and sensitivity to insulin. When we sleep during the day, it can throw off our body's natural rhythms.

Ayurveda views napping as an activity that increases kapha, and all types of type 2 diabetes start as a kapha imbalance. Western medicine has several theories to explain the relationship between napping and the risk of type 2 diabetes. Napping raises glucose levels and alters metabolism, increases insulin secretion, produces inflammation and stress hormones, as well as disrupts circadian rhythms and increases the risk of morbidity. For those who are pre-diabetic or concerned about their blood glucose, getting a good night's sleep will go a long way toward helping the body use insulin efficiently. Getting 6 to 7 hours of sleep at night, avoiding daytime napping, reducing sedentary behavior, increasing daily steps, and including a regular exercise routine are key to preventing or reversing type 2 diabetes.

Three Tools to Silence Stress

Stress is another critical factor in developing type 2 diabetes, and many people with this condition suffer from diabetes-related distress. General emotional stress, anxiety, anger, depression, and hostility increase the risk for developing type 2 diabetes. During times of stress, the body goes through three stages: the alarm phase (fight or flight), the resistance phase (in which resistance to the stress builds), and the exhaustion phase (when the duration of stress is sufficiently long). The body becomes familiar with this process and anticipates a response to stress by making physiological changes. We experience stress at all levels—cognitive, emotional, physical, and behavioral, leading to a wide variety of symptoms such as poor judgment, anger, anxiety, diarrhea, nausea, increased heart rate, and elevated blood glucose.

Emotional stress can increase the risk of developing type 2 diabetes in different ways. Chronic stress reactions are due to long-term activation of the adrenal glands and the sympathetic nervous system. When under any kind of stress, such as a blood-sugar crash or daily stress, the body produces degenerative stress-fighting hormones called cortisol and adrenaline. These hormones enter the bloodstream and increase respiratory rates. The body automatically directs blood to the limbs and muscles, preparing you for physical action—fight or flight. Today, stress is most likely a response to a psychological or emotional cause rather than a physical danger, so the body does not use the blood glucose in the limbs for energy. If the body does not physically convert glucose into energy, blood glucose levels become elevated.

Another problem occurs when cortisol and adrenaline are released, which causes the body to store fat. When the body gets accustomed to receiving its energy this way, weight gain happens more easily. We tend to overeat when we have a blood sugar crash, and then fat storage continues during stress and as a response to stress recovery.

Cortisol also triggers sugar cravings because the body can use sugar and carbs instantly as fuel instead of fat. Under pressure, we tend to make poor decisions. After a stressful day, it's easy to eat simple carbs, skip a workout, and have a cigarette or cocktail.

Excessive stress has other adverse effects on the body. It irritates the mucous membrane of the intestines, compromising detoxification and nutrient metabolism. It also slows down a healthy immune response and the body's natural detox pathways. Trillions of microbes, which support immunity and bodily functions, are damaged with the inflammatory stress response in the mucosal lining of the gut, which can also lead to diarrhea, constipation, and inflammatory bowel diseases.

Stress causes a chain reaction of events that compromise the body's ability to lose weight, balance blood sugar, properly digest food, and eliminate waste. Stress is a contributing factor to many cases of type 2 diabetes. People who experience a significant life event such as a divorce, financial distress, or the loss of a job are nearly twice as likely to develop type 2 diabetes. These people in particular need to include stress reduction as part of their wellness program. Ayurveda provides many well-researched and supported tools to reduce stress and reverse type 2 diabetes.

Tool #1: Yoga

Yoga, a mindfulness practice that emphasizes relaxation, meditation, and deep breathing, is particularly beneficial for people with type 2 diabetes. It has existed for thousands of years and can easily be incorporated into your lifestyle. It is simple for people of all ages to learn. Classes are widely available in many communities, and it requires little equipment. Once trained, people can practice at home, making it a low-cost tool for reducing stress and improving type 2 diabetes.

Yoga reduces stress and balances the mind for complete physical, mental, and spiritual health. It teaches the fundamental principle of unity between mind, body, and spirit. If the mind is stressed or agitated, the health of the body becomes compromised. If the body is in poor health, emotional strength and mental clarity are negatively affected.

A regular yoga practice positively impacts movement and supports healthy decision-making that contribute to improved glycemic control. When we feel good, we make better decisions about our health. Yoga is one of the tools that helps us feel good, both physically and mentally. The yoga poses recommended for stress-induced type 2 diabetes are gentle and restorative. Yoga includes both mindful movement and mental relaxation. This approach works to manage type 2 diabetes since mindfulness training increases one's ability to recognize and effectively respond to and cope with emotional stress. People with type 2 diabetes who practice yoga experience lower stress levels after a class. Yoga prevents stress-induced rises in cortisol, thus controlling the increase in blood glucose levels. Reducing stress improves mindfulness, and having a regular yoga practice may help you become more tuned into your health and wellness. Daily practice leads to improved self-care behaviors, including diet and lifestyle choices.

Numerous research studies support the use of yoga for glycemic control among patients with type 2 diabetes. Researchers have found that yoga stimulates insulin production. The various movements in a yoga practice massage the internal organs. Forward bends massage the pancreas and increase insulin production. Twisted poses put pressure on the intestines and help move waste through the colon, and inversions improve circulation.

Yoga has been shown to reduce blood glucose and cholesterol levels in just 9 days. Yoga can also improve insulin sensitivity and reduce oxidative stress.

The yoga poses included later in this book have been proven through clinical research to help balance type 2 diabetes.

Tool #2: Meditation

People recently diagnosed with type 2 diabetes may experience substantial stress. The difficulty of implementing the recommended changes in diet and lifestyle, as well as the worry about diabetes-related complications, can become overwhelming. Some people may find themselves living in unhelpful environments. Without support from friends and family, making these changes may feel especially challenging. Feeling unsupported and overwhelmed can negatively affect their perception of their future, resulting in despair, hopelessness, and powerlessness. These negative beliefs have an impact on self-care, diet, exercise, and blood sugar testing. It is therefore crucial for people with type 2 diabetes to find a supportive community and practice meditation for stress management.

Meditation is particularly useful in the early stages of diagnosis because this is when you might experience the most stress and anxiety. Meditation helps reduce negative thoughts, thereby preventing the onset of anxiety and mood disorders, which can complicate type 2 diabetes management and self-care. Meditation allows the mind and body to become present and relaxed. The body's energies can run freely, permitting the body to heal itself and the mind to teach itself. Meditation causes changes in the brain that help control responses to stress. People with a regular meditation practice are therefore less prone to stress.

Creating a Daily Meditation Practice

Creating a daily meditation practice can release cyclical thinking and stuck emotions, allowing you to tap into your authentic, best self. Every meditation practice is unique to the individual. There is no right or wrong way to meditate, but here are a few key concepts you may wish to include in your practice:

1. Set an intention. Start by thinking about the purpose of your practice. What is your motivation? Stress reduction? Improving mental clarity? Reducing negative thought patterns? Having a healthy motivation will draw you into your practice and align your purpose with other elements of your health and wellness program.

2. Determine a regular time that fits into your lifestyle. Traditionally, meditation times were based on solar cycles. Ayurvedic rishis practiced meditation in the morning before sunrise, when the universe is still and present. Find a time in your schedule when you are free from interruptions. Choose a consistent time to make meditation part of your daily routine. For some people, this may mean getting up 15 minutes earlier in the morning so that they have some private time before everyone else in the house is awake. For others, it may mean leaving

for work 15 minutes earlier so that they can have some uninterrupted time in a parked car before going into work. Please do not attempt to meditate while driving. A parked vehicle, however, can be peaceful and quiet.

Before bed, meditation relaxes the mind and prepares us for sleep. In the morning, it clears the mind and prepares us for the day. The time you choose is up to you, but it should be a consistent time with no phones, foods, drinks, or people to distract you.

3. Choose a place that is quiet and free from disturbances. Create a meditation space by decorating it with items that are meaningful to you. You may include objects that deepen your practice while aligning you closer with your intention. Choose things that inspire you to relax and meditate, such as pillows, essential oils, crystals, music, or candles.

4. Settle in. Once you have set your intention and chosen your time and place, it's time to settle into your practice. Spend the first few minutes getting comfortable and preparing for the meditation. Preparing for meditation will enable you to completely and fully benefit from the time spent in meditation. Start by finding a comfortable seated position and gently soften or close your eyes. Take one hand and place it on your belly. Feel your hand move outward with the inhales and gently pull inward with the exhales.

Gradually scan your body from head to toe to find any tension. Consciously relax the muscles throughout your body. Contract and release, or gently massage, any areas of the body where you feel discomfort. Start with your forehead and feel the relaxation spread through your body down your neck, shoulders, arms, chest, abdomen, hips, thighs, knees, calves, ankles, and to your feet. You may feel warmth, heaviness, tingling, or floating as signs of relaxation. Some people may feel nothing specific.

5. Start to meditate. During the meditation, you can use a word or an image as a focal point to control your auditory and visual senses. The word you choose should be positive, one that brings you back to your intention without any intense emotional energy attached to it. Words such as *peace, love, om, one,* or *relax* work well. Some people find it easier to say their word with their breath. You can also use the rise and fall of your abdomen as you breathe, repeating the word *inhale* as you inhale and *exhale* as you release.

You can also choose a visual symbol such as a candle, a rising sun, something in nature, or an abstract design. With your eyes half-closed, focus on the symbol and repeat your chosen word. After several minutes, gently close your eyes fully and visualize the symbol and repeat the word in your head. After a few more minutes, imagine the symbol and sound merging and dissolving into space. When you have a distracting thought or vision, recognize it without judgment and label it as a thought. Then open your eyes, bring your attention back to your visual symbol, begin repeating your word again, and slowly bring yourself back into the meditative state. The goal is to recognize thought patterns, reduce mental chatter, and create mental space. The sooner we can identify negative thought patterns, the quicker we can correct them and enter into peace of mind. The first days of practicing meditation are the most difficult, but stick with it. Meditation becomes more natural, less forced, and a state of mind throughout your day.

Guided meditations and timers are fantastic tools to use when starting a meditation practice. Meditating on your own requires some effort, while guided meditations walk you through a meditation and help you find a calm and peaceful state one step at a time. There are many apps available that you can use. A meditation class with an instructor can provide additional support, answer any questions you may have, and help you overcome obstacles. You will also find specific meditations based on your constitution later in this book.

Tool #3: Breathwork

Of the three stress reduction tools, breathwork is perhaps the quickest and easiest way to calm the mind and relax the body. In Ayurveda, *prana* is the energetic flow of the breath and the vital life force that runs throughout the body. Breathing is an automatic function; it happens without having to think about it. But when our conscious mind controls the breath, significant emotional changes occur. Breathing is the bridge to consciousness. By mindfully focusing on the breath, we can melt away our external world and find calm, inner peace.

The breath is a physiological function that we can control. And when our breath is slow and deep, we can reduce our heart rate. According to Ayurveda, there is a deep connection between the heart and the mind. The heart is the seat of love and compassion, and, through deep breathing, we can increase positive emotions in our heart. The heart secretes neuropeptides that are responsible for processing thoughts, feelings, and emotions. When we get out of balance, neuropeptides produce symptoms related to anxiety. When we are in balance, neuropeptides produce messages that help us become calm and happy. Deepening the breath increases the production of neuropeptides that keep us in a balanced state. Breathing practices are therefore essential for managing stress, cardiovascular health, and type 2 diabetes.

The breath is closely connected with the mind, making breathwork a perfect mind/body practice that anyone can use during times of stress. A few minutes of focused breathwork releases tension and transitions the mind and body into a refreshed state. Stress hormones decrease, pancreatic functions return to normal, and we feel a sense of well-being. By slowing the breath and observing its rhythm, we turn our attention inward and reconnect to our inner strength. Regulated breathing practices improve sleep, relieve stress, decrease heart rate, calm nervous energy, manage pain, enhance digestion, and improve concentration. Research also indicates that Ayurvedic breathing exercises can reduce blood glucose levels in people with type 2 diabetes.

Conscious regulation of the breath influences brain functioning. When the breath is steady and deep, the mind will follow and become centered and quiet. Neuro-respiratory integration occurs when the breath and the brain connect—practicing deep belly breathing throughout the day is a sure way to calm the nervous system.

Slow, meditative breathing also works to prepare the body for a good night's sleep. Deep belly breathing stimulates pineal gland function, which increases melatonin levels. Melatonin is a powerful hormone that reduces stress and promotes good quality sleep. People who practice breathwork can increase their melatonin levels by up to 10 times.

We can attribute breathwork's powerful effects to its ability to influence ultradian rhythms. Ultradian rhythms are cycles that control the desire to eat and drink, actions of the immune system, hormone secretions, stress reactions, concentration ability, and mood changes. These physiological functions are all governed by the same 90 to 120–minute cycles as our breathing, and breathwork helps to normalize these rhythms.

We breathe through one nostril at a time, for about 90 to 120 minutes, then breathe through both nostrils for 20 minutes, and then breathe through the other nostril for another 90 to 120 minutes. We are unconscious of this rhythm, yet it occurs continuously throughout our life. When we breathe through our right nostril, the left hemisphere of our brain is more active. The left side of our brain is responsible for linear thinking, assertiveness, concentrated study, and logical problem solving. Right nostril breathing stimulates the sympathetic nervous system, increasing blood pressure, alertness, and readiness for action, preparing us for intense physical activity or assertive exchanges. If you are feeling tired and mentally sluggish during the day, plug your left nostril and breathe through your right nostril for a few minutes. Right nostril breathing will allow you to regain focus and energy.

Left nostril breathing activates the right side of our brain, which cultivates creativity, intuition, non-linear thinking, artistic skills, and musical talent. Left nostril breathing activates the parasympathetic nervous system. Left nostril breathing reduces blood pressure, promotes healthy digestion and elimination, reduces stress hormones, and increases relaxation.

During the 20 minutes when both nostrils are actively breathing, the mind and body are more integrated. Mentally we feel present and mindful of the body's signals. We can acknowledge emotional states with fewer adverse reactions, and we feel centered and calm.

Here are some helpful tips to establish a breathwork practice:

- Find a comfortable seated position.
- Sit with a straight spine.
- Put your feet flat on the floor, about hip-width apart.
- Relax your stomach muscles, allowing you to take longer, fuller, deeper breaths.
- Rest your hands on your belly.

Grounding is essential for breathwork. Give yourself a few minutes to allow your mind to become aware of your breath. Notice your breath. At first, it may feel fast and shallow; this is normal. Become aware of how your body feels with each breath. Breathe into any tension or discomfort. Be kind to yourself and allow your body to relax as you settle into your rhythm.

Breathe in and out through your nose. Inhales and exhales should feel natural. As you inhale, allow your belly to balloon out, filling with new air. As you exhale, gently engage your abdominal muscles. Do not push yourself to take slow or long inhales and exhales. The flow of breath is a cycle of inhaling, pausing, exhaling, pausing, and so on. The transition into the pauses is smooth. Don't hold your breath at any time.

Practice filtering out the sounds of the external world by shifting your focus to the internal sound of your breath. Your thoughts are energy. Let your energy flow through your breath. Once you notice a nice rhythm and feel your body and mind relaxing, you are there. If your attention starts to drift, bring your focus back to the sound of your breathing. Ayurveda offers unique breathing practices for vata, pitta, and kapha people. Yoga, breathwork, and meditation are critical components of this 12-week program.

Herbal Therapies

Plants have provided medicinal support to millions of people for thousands of years. The majority of people living in developing countries rely on herbal medicine as their primary form of healthcare. Today, humankind continues to better understand the value of herbs, as scientific research and new discoveries reveal their valuable antidiabetic properties. Plants are a magnificent source of bioactive compounds and can help balance many different health conditions including type 2 diabetes.

Herbs are a source of compounds that are used to formulate pharmaceutical drugs. The popular antidiabetic drug metformin was isolated from *Galega officinalis,* an herb commonly known as goat's rue. However, when single-plant compounds are isolated and used for drug manufacturing, it produces many of the pharmaceutical side effects. Many oral antidiabetic drugs fail to give long-term glycemic control and have limited usage due to their side effects. Herbal therapies, on the other hand, have antidiabetic properties that help lower blood glucose, with minimal or no side effects.

There is a vital quest to discover herbal antidiabetic solutions, and Ayurveda has a long and promising history of herbal therapies for type 2 diabetes. Many single herbs and polyherbal formulations are available. Neem, *Gymnema sylvestre,* and tulsi are just a few single herbs that are widely available and known for their beneficial effects. Chandraprabha vati, ayaskriti, and triphala are polyherbal Ayurvedic formulas that are also very effective for type 2 diabetes.

Single Herbs

Neem *(Azadirachta indica)*
The incredible neem tree was declared the "tree of the twenty-first century" by the United Nations. Neem has had more than 4,000 years of use in Ayurveda. For centuries, millions of people have cleaned their teeth with neem twigs, treated skin disorders with neem leaf juice, taken neem tea as a tonic, and placed neem leaves in grain bins, cupboards, and closets to keep pesky bugs away. Neem has many healing actions that help relieve pain, reduce infections, and eliminate parasites. Indian people have long revered the neem tree and employed all its parts for medicinal and household uses. Neem acts as a "village pharmacy" to millions of people in India, and practitioners of modern medicine are now advocating neem as a valuable herb for treating type 2 diabetes.

The medicinal properties of neem are in the fruit, seeds, oil, leaves, roots, and bark. Both neem leaf and seed have demonstrated hypoglycemic effects. The leaf is slightly more effective than the seed oil; the leaf has been shown to significantly reduce blood glucose after a few weeks of regular administration. Neem's light, bitter, and astringent qualities, along with its pungent post-digestive effect, reduce the heaviness associated with kapha. The light quality, however, can aggravate vata. The external skin of neem is astringent, and the internal composition is pungent.

The chemical composition of neem makes it useful for alleviating type 2 diabetes. The bioactive compounds are responsible for neem's hypoglycemic effects and bitter taste. These compounds open glucose pathways, thus increasing peripheral glucose uptake and reducing blood sugar.

Neem decreases blood glucose spikes related to both dietary intake and stress. When we react to stress, the adrenal glands secrete adrenaline, which causes the liver to release stored glucose into the bloodstream, creating high blood sugar. If stress occurs regularly and the major muscle groups are not activated to promote glucose uptake, type 2 diabetes can develop. Adrenaline is an essential contributor to stress-induced hyperglycemia, increasing the risk of type 2 diabetes. Neem is ideal for both dietary and stress-related causes of hyperglycemia.

Many well-implemented studies, as well as traditional observational Ayurvedic studies, have demonstrated the value of neem as a treatment for type 2 diabetes.

Sardunika/Gurmar/Madhuharini *(Gymnema sylvestre)*

Gymnema sylvestre is commonly known as sardunika, gurmar, or madhuharini in Ayurveda. It is a multi-branch, broad-growing herb with long, oval leaves and yellow flowers. The leaves contain resin, gymnemic acid, tartaric acid, and enzymes that help balance type 2 diabetes.

Internally, *Gymnema sylvestre* works mainly on the digestive system. It has light, rough, and astringent qualities that reduce blood sugar by acting on the pancreas, adrenal glands, and digestive organs. *Gymnema sylvestre* assists with insulin secretions from the pancreas and repairs the pancreas. It can balance fasting blood glucose levels within 20 days. Once restored, the pancreas can produce more insulin to stabilize glucose in the blood and urine. This makes *Gymnema sylvestre* very helpful for treating type 2 diabetes.

Gymnema sylvestre is known as the "sugar destroyer" in Ayurveda because it has the unique ability to modify the taste of sweet things, thereby reducing cravings for sweets. It helps balance blood glucose by regenerating pancreatic cells, reducing the need for prescription medication. One study found that more than 20 percent of patients were able to discontinue prescription drug use and balance blood glucose with *Gymnema sylv*estre alone.

Obesity is commonly associated with type 2 diabetes, and *Gymnema sylvestre* assists in weight loss. It works by reducing insulin resistance and oxidative stress, among other actions. It also offers cardiac protection by increasing cellular functions and maintaining the structure of the muscles of the heart.

Tulsi *(Ocimum sanctum L.)*

Ayurveda uses *Ocimum sanctum L.,* commonly known as tulsi or holy basil, for its diverse healing properties. Tulsi is a sacred and cherished herb found in many homes across India. Marked by its strong aroma and astringent taste, it is regarded in Ayurveda as an "elixir of life" and is believed to promote longevity. Tulsi increases physical endurance and helps the body handle stress.

Tulsi balances type 2 diabetes through its ability to reduce inflammation. Chronic inflammation is associated with metabolic syndrome and increased risk of type 2 diabetes. Tulsi excels at reducing both acute and chronic inflammation. Compounds in tulsi exhibit both antioxidant and anti-inflammatory properties. The potent anti-inflammatory effects of tulsi are comparable to nonsteroidal anti-inflammatory drugs, such as ibuprofen and aspirin.

Many studies have found that tulsi improves blood glucose, lipids, and blood pressure in people with type 2 diabetes. One study found that tulsi improved fasting blood glucose in 90 percent of patients. Others have also found that daily ingestion of tulsi leaves produces a dramatic decrease in fasting blood glucose, postprandial (post-meal) glucose, and urine glucose in patients with type 2 diabetes. Tulsi has also been shown to lower markers of poor cardiovascular health within 12 weeks. It accomplishes these healing actions by reducing inflammation and free-radical damage in the liver, kidneys, and pancreas. With less damage and inflammation, organ function improves, and the pancreas produces insulin more efficiently. More efficient insulin production increases cellular glucose uptake, reducing blood glucose levels.

Tulsi works together with medications and other herbs. When used as a combined therapy with the antidiabetic drug glibenclamide (Glyburide), tulsi improves blood glucose better than drug treatment alone. Tulsi has a synergistic effect when used in combination with other herbs and produces a more significant reduction in type 2 diabetes symptoms. The most notable effect occurs when used with neem. Tulsi is ideal for reversing type 2 diabetes. It lowers fasting blood glucose, post-meal glucose, chronic inflammation, and unhealthy fats when administered for 12 weeks.

Herbal Formulations

Medicinal herbs contain thousands of unique plant compounds that promote healing in numerous ways. Many of the medical benefits of plants have not been investigated through clinical research but indicated through thousands of years of observational studies. Synergy is a fundamental concept in herbal medicine. It occurs in multi-herbal formulas when the effect of one herb improves the healing potential of another. Herbal synergy occurs when phytochemicals become more bioavailable. For example, when turmeric is combined with black pepper, turmeric's active compound curcumin increases by as much as 2,000 percent.

Formulating herbs together increases the availability of some plant compounds and alters the absorption of others. Synergistic actions reduce side effects and can increase safety, as you can take much less and get more benefits than you would with a single herb. Triphala, chandraprabha vati, and ayaskriti are three herbal formulas that Ayurveda uses to balance type 2 diabetes.

Triphala: The Three Fruits

Triphala is a rejuvenating formula used frequently in Ayurveda. The classic text *Charaka Samhita* describes triphala as a regenerating tonic that gives energy, supports strength, and increases immunity. Triphala can be used in all stages of life, from childhood through old age. Its therapeutic effects work to balance and revitalize vata, pitta, and kapha. Triphala has a unique quality that balances all doshas and constitutions.

Triphala consists of equal portions of three medicinal herbs: amalaki (*Emblica officinalis gaertn.*), haritaki (*Terminalia chebula retz.*), and bibhitaki (Terminalia bellerica gaertn.). Ayurvedic pharmacology describes the taste of triphala as sweet, sour, pungent, bitter, and astringent. The classic text *Astanga Hrdayam* refers to triphala as the "best rejuvenator of the body, cures diseases of the eyes, heals wounds and cure skin diseases, excess moisture of the tissues, obesity, diabetes, aggravation of kapha and asra [blood]." From ancient to modern times, a variety of formulations have used triphala.

Triphala continues to grow in popularity as a treatment for type 2 diabetes. It has been shown to reduce weight, balance blood sugar, and have other antidiabetic effects when used for 12 weeks. Triphala acts similarly to prescription drugs. It decreases the absorption of glucose by inhibiting the process enzymes use to convert starch into glucose. This process can ultimately predispose a person to high blood glucose levels. Experts therefore believe that impeding the digestive process of starch could play a vital role in the management of type 2 diabetes.

Current drugs such as acarbose (Precose), voglibose (Volix), and miglitol (Glyset) also inhibit these enzymes. However, they produce side effects such as abdominal discomfort and diarrhea. The plant compounds in triphala inhibit the activity of these enzymes without the debilitating side effects.

Through triphala's ability to inhibit enzymes, it protects people with diabetes and those predisposed to it. Elevated blood glucose can cause severe damage through glycation, in which sugar molecules bind to protein molecules in the body, which can lead to nerve damage or blindness. The tannins present in triphala inhibit the process of glycation, reducing blood glucose levels.

Triphala also promotes healthy digestion. It reduces sluggishness, abdominal pain, inflammation, and indigestion, and it detoxifies the digestive tract. Triphala helps treat type 2 diabetes, as well as obesity and other diseases of oversaturation. Modern medical science has found that it decreases glucose absorption, inhibits glycation, reduces weight, and performs other actions related to metabolic disorders.

Chandraprabha Vati: Glowing Moon

Chandraprabha vati brings a calm vitality to the body. Chandraprabha means "glowing moon," as it imparts a rejuvenated radiance. As a revitalizing health tonic, chandraprabha vati reduces general weakness and increases physical strength. It also alleviates stress, leaving the body relaxed and refreshed.

The most renowned Ayurvedic texts on herbal preparations highly recommend chandraprabha vati as an excellent remedy for type 2 diabetes. Chandraprabha vati promotes the healthy functioning of the kidneys by reducing abnormal sugar content in the urine and reducing frequent urination. This classic Ayurvedic formula also helps with diabetes-related complications such as abdominal distension, colicky pain, cysts, anemia, painful urination, kidney stones, hemorrhoids, urinary obstruction, hernia, lower back pain, skin diseases, itching, tastelessness, impaired digestion, and weakness.

Chandraprabha vati has shown remarkable promise in treating obesity, metabolic syndrome, and type 2 diabetes. It contains 37 herbs, most of which have glucose- and lipid-reducing abilities. Research supports the use of chandraprabha vati to reduce glucose, cholesterol, and triglyceride levels. It produces comparable effects to metformin. Chandraprabha vati causes molecular changes, which contribute to its antidiabetic and anti-inflammatory effects.

I strongly advise anyone interested in trying chandraprabha vati to consult with a certified Ayurvedic practitioner before taking it. Your practitioner can help you find the ideal dosage for your constitution. Excessive consumption may lead to ulcerative colitis, stomach ulcers, or a burning sensation in the abdomen. Chandraprabha vati is contraindicated for those with a blood disorder known as thalassemia. People suffering from hypertension should only take this medicine only after a thorough consultation, as it contains salt.

Ayaskriti: Iron Out the Kinks

Ayaskriti is an herbal formulation that is effective at balancing type 2 diabetes and its related complications. *Ayas* in Sanskrit means "iron," and the herbal formulation includes medicinal herbs and metallic iron. Oxidative stress contributes to insulin resistance and the development of type 2 diabetes. A person with this disease is in a chronic state of hyperglycemia, which promotes glycation and the formation of free radicals. These free radicals cause the vascular complications found in type 2 diabetes. Inhibiting the creation of free radicals therefore prevents oxidative stress and related complications.

The antioxidant properties found in ayaskriti help explain its effectiveness. Antioxidants act in different ways; some inhibit the formation of free radicals, while others increase the defensive capabilities of enzymes, thereby protecting tissues. Research has indicated that the antioxidant activity of the herbal compounds in ayaskriti helps treat type 2 diabetes. Ayaskriti reduces many of the symptoms of type 2 diabetes, such as:

- Frequent urination
- Cloudy urine
- Sweet taste in the mouth
- Increased hunger
- Burning sensation in the hands and feet
- Numbness in the hands and feet
- Lassitude
- Increased perspiration
- Excessive sleeping

Ayaskriti reduces fasting blood glucose and post-meal blood glucose. A dose of 25 ml of ayaskriti, twice daily after food for 30 days, helps manage type 2 diabetes without any known adverse reactions.

As with chandraprabha vati, I strongly advise anyone interested in using ayaskriti to consult with a certified Ayurvedic practitioner before taking it. This will help you find the best dosage for your constitution and prevent potential side effects. When there is an increase in pitta, ayaskriti can cause hyperacidity and excessive heat.

Ayurvedic Detoxification: Panchakarma

For thousands of years, Ayurveda's remedies have proven their effectiveness. Detoxification plays a pivotal role in Ayurveda's preventive, curative, and rehabilitative powers for type 2 diabetes. Panchakarma is a deep purification treatment, vital for correcting this condition. The umbrella of panchakarma includes five major therapeutic procedures: vamana (therapeutic vomiting), virechana (therapeutic purgation), basti (therapeutic enema), rakta moksha (therapeutic bloodletting), and nasya (therapeutic nose drops). It also includes many other applied therapies to support the five main procedures. In the US, however, we do not practice vamana or rakta moksha. We will focus on virechana because it is the most influential procedure in working with type 2 diabetes.

Panchakarma not only works as a treatment for type 2 diabetes, but it also plays an essential role in prevention and management. Panchakarma improves digestive strength, which helps treat the disease. The purification procedures used in panchakarma naturally remove stagnation, imbalanced doshas, and toxins from the body, so it works far beyond glucose control to manage type 2 diabetes. Virechana pulls the imbalanced doshas from the deep tissues, into the digestive tract, and out of the body.

Virechana Purification

Virechana successfully reduces both fasting blood sugar and post-meal blood sugar by lowering glucose production in the liver. Virechana, as a panchakarma procedure, balances the doshas. And when used for type 2 diabetes, it improves glucose metabolism on a cellular level and alleviates pitta-dominant symptoms such as nerve damage and excessive sweating. Purgatives eliminate pitta from the liver, gallbladder, and small intestine. This helps the body decongest bile, remove obstructions that inhibit metabolism and digestion, and function more efficiently. Studies demonstrate that virechana improves the digestive fire, promotes proper elimination, removes unhealthy gut flora, improves sleep patterns, reduces heaviness in the abdomen, and decreases LDL and total cholesterol.

Virechana eliminates toxic substances such as metabolic waste, mucus, and excess doshas from the body to promote health and immunity. Waste substances are removed from the digestive tract through specific procedures and are eliminated through bowel movements. Virechana works because it extracts the materials that create blockages in the body, allowing for a smooth flow of energy. After cleansing, the body's metabolism increases, and insulin resistance reduces. Metabolic waste is a dense, slimy, sticky substance produced through impaired digestion. Water, fat, and toxic substances are all part of metabolic waste. The body has many channels of elimination to remove these substances from the body. The kidneys and sweat glands remove water-soluble toxins. The liver and digestive system remove fat-soluble toxins. Panchakarma uses internal oleation to help remove fat-soluble toxins. Oils such as ghee or flaxseed oil are used to gently soften the bond between the fat-soluble toxins and delicate tissues. In doing so, they extract toxins without injuring the body.

Molecules move from a higher concentration to a lower concentration when separated by a diffusible membrane. The mucosal lining of the gastrointestinal tract is a perfect example of such a membrane. Concentrated toxic molecules move from the body's tissues through the mucosal lining, into the digestive tract, and into the ghee or flaxseed oil. Virechana removes mucus, decaying red blood cells, damaged white blood cells, unhealthy epithelial cells, and parasites, which inhibit metabolic function and immunity. Therefore, it is essential to remove these toxic substances in the treatment of type 2 diabetes.

Virechana effectively treats many of the symptoms of type 2 diabetes—frequent urination, cloudy urine, indigestion, obesity—and it balances unhealthy fats. It also reduces symptoms like burning of the hands and feet, extreme hunger, stickiness in the mouth, and cramps. Virechana also successfully reduces both fasting blood sugar and post-meal blood sugar. Virechana corrects blockages in the body by extracting corrupted doshas and metabolic waste. It is this cleansing action that reduces insulin resistance.

Classic Ayurvedic texts state that virechana should produce the following results:

- Removing blockages that inhibit the downward flow of vata in the pelvis
- Refreshing the sense organs
- Lightening the body
- Eliminating excess doshas

In one study, 88 percent of participants who used panchakarma procedures experienced lightness in the body, and more than half of the participants experienced all of the above results. Virechana works by removing blockages, which allows vata to flow freely. When vata can move freely, you will experience feelings of lightness and clarity. This makes it beneficial for the treatment of type 2 diabetes, as well as many other kapha imbalances.

Panchakarma treatment should be the first line of therapy for obesity and type 2 diabetes. Ayurvedic theory states that the disease process begins with digestion. When digestion is out of balance, absorption diminishes, and waste accumulates. In one study, 76 percent of participants experienced an increase in digestive strength after virechana, thereby correcting the root cause of the imbalance.

Balancing digestion helps the body metabolize herbal medicines. When we administer Ayurvedic herbs orally, they first go to the stomach. If there is metabolic waste in the stomach, the herbs are not properly digested and used by the body. Metabolic waste dampens the digestive fire, hindering the body's ability to metabolize herbs. With the help of virechana, cleansing occurs, digestion and absorption normalize, and the body can receive the full benefits of herbal supplements. Virechana, when used in conjunction with herbal formulas, relieves excess urination, balances unhealthy fats, alleviates extreme hunger, improves cloudy urine, and reduces laziness and excessive sweating.

In many ways, panchakarma is more effective than modern pharmaceutical medicine in treating type 2 diabetes. One research study designed to compare the effects of panchakarma and dietary changes against metformin demonstrated impressive results for Ayurvedic therapies. The panchakarma procedures showed encouraging results in improving metabolism and overall well-being in people with prediabetes. The panchakarma and dietary-intervention group showed a significant reduction in glucose and lipid levels. Panchakarma also improved many symptoms such as extreme thirst, dryness in the mouth, burning sensation, laziness, extreme hunger, excessive sleep, and frequent urination. Dietary changes and panchakarma corrected more symptoms than metformin, as the metformin group only experienced a significant improvement in frequent urination.

According to the *Charaka Samhita*, "Just as silt develops surely over time, even in pure water kept undisturbed in an earthen pot, so also dirt accumulates inside the body, so one should undergo detoxification." Regular detoxification is essential for preventing type 2 diabetes. By removing the cause of the disease and undergoing seasonal cleansing, we remove waste from the body so that it does not accumulate and contribute to type 2 diabetes.

CHAPTER 4

THE 12-WEEK PROGRAM: INTRODUCTION

Program Structure

- Part I: 8-Week Constitution and Elimination Diet
- Part II: 1-Week Detox and Restoration
- Part III: 3-Week Rebuilding and Reintroduction of Foods

Cultivating Support

Successful completion of this program relies on having community support. Research shows that it's much easier for us to reach our health goals if we have a few allies. I encourage you to let your family and friends know about *The Ayurveda Solution for Type 2 Diabetes.* Ask people to join you on your walking, resistance training, and exercise program. It's much easier to stay motivated when you have a workout partner or trainer. Have people join you in meal preparation, teach the recipes to others, and host blood-sugar-balancing dinner parties so you can enjoy the meals together.

Creating Your Routine for Success

Success in this program means creating a regular routine and sticking to it. You will likely be incorporating some major changes into your daily schedule over the next 12 weeks. The recommended mealtimes and sleep schedules are very important for balancing hormones, reducing stress, and minimizing blood sugar spikes.

Try planning your day in advance by following the recommended bedtime. Using the bedtime as an anchor will give you the right amount of sleep you need to feel well-rested, and you will be ready to get up at the recommended wake time. Waking early in the morning will give you plenty of time to get your morning exercise in, and you will be hungry at the recommended mealtimes. Going to bed early also helps you avoid any late-night snacking, which can cause your fasting blood glucose levels to be high.

Biometric Goal Setting

Biometrics, or body measurements and calculations, are a great way to track your improvements. One example is BMI. Body mass index (BMI) is a value that represents the ratio of a person's weight to their height. BMI may be used to estimate body fat and a person's risk for diseases that can occur from excess body fat. The higher your BMI, the higher your risk for certain diseases such as type 2 diabetes. Use a BMI calculator to determine your BMI. If your BMI is 25 or higher, your weight-loss goal is 7 percent of your total body weight.

Self-Monitoring Your Blood Sugar

Throughout the program, it's important to regularly monitor your blood sugar. Self-monitoring will prevent blood glucose from getting too high or too low. Knowing your blood glucose level can also help you adjust your dietary intake, physical activity, and insulin doses as needed.

Blood sugar testing requires the use of a blood glucose meter, called a glucometer. The meter measures the amount of sugar in a small sample of blood, usually from a pinprick on your fingertip, which you place on a disposable test strip. Test results are recorded in a logbook or stored in the glucose meter's electronic memory. Your healthcare provider may recommend an appropriate device for you. He or she can also teach you how to use your meter, or you can follow the instructions that come with it. In general, here's how the process works:

1. Wash and dry your hands well. (Food and other substances on your fingers can give an inaccurate reading.)
2. Insert a test strip into your meter.
3. Wipe the area you plan to prick with an alcohol wipe and allow the alcohol to dry completely.
4. Prick the side of your fingertip with the needle (lancet) provided with your test kit.
5. Touch and hold the edge of the test strip to the drop of blood.
6. The meter will display your blood sugar level on a screen after a few seconds.

The frequency with which people with type 2 diabetes should monitor their blood glucose level varies. Non-insulin dependent diabetics should monitor blood glucose three times a day—preferably fasting blood glucose, which is measured in the morning before eating or drinking, 2 hours after the heaviest meal, and before going to bed. People who use insulin should measure their blood glucose as instructed by their healthcare provider.

As you begin monitoring your blood glucose, you will find that your range is higher than the goal. Do not become frustrated—as you implement the program, you will see a reduction in your blood glucose. Pay close attention to your blood glucose numbers so that they stay within the recommended range and do not get too low. Work closely with your healthcare provider to make any necessary adjustments in your medications.

Blood Glucose Goals:
- Fasting/waking: 85–120
- 2 hours after meals: 100–140
- Before bed: 100–140

Use the journal below to track your blood sugar throughout the 12-week program. Today, you are in the "Start" column. Write down your waking blood glucose and two post-meal blood glucose readings. Also, record your weight and BMI. You will find a link to a BMI calculator in the resources section on page 183. If your BMI is 25 or higher, your weight-loss goal is 7 percent of your total weight. To fill out the "Hip and Waist Circumferences" row, use a tape measure to measure the smallest part of your waist, then measure the widest part of your hips. Record your hip and waist circumferences. Throughout this program, take three blood glucose readings per day. Record those numbers in the appropriate column for each week. At the end of each week, weigh yourself, determine your BMI, measure your hip and waist circumferences, and write those numbers in the journal. I also recommend taking a picture of yourself each week to document the changes. It's very encouraging to see before and after pictures!

Biometric Journal to Track Your Success

	Start	Wk. 1	Wk. 2	Wk. 3	Wk. 4	Wk. 5	Wk. 6	Wk. 7	Wk. 8	Wk. 9	Wk. 10	Wk. 11	Wk. 12
Waking Blood Glucose													
2 hr. Post-Meal Blood Glucose													
Before Bed Blood Glucose													
Weight and BMI													
Hip and Waist Circumference													

CHAPTER 5

The 12-Week Program: Starting the 8-Week Constitution and Elimination Diet

Identifying Dietary Guidelines

It is important to remember that we are all unique and come to the table with our digestive strengths and weaknesses. If there are any foods that do not "agree" with you, please exclude them throughout the program. For example, if you know that dairy makes you feel bloated, please avoid it. It's also important to eliminate any foods you eat every day. When you consume a certain food on a daily basis, your body can develop a sensitivity or allergy to it, so it's important to rotate new foods into the diet. If there are any foods on the list for your constitution that you consume daily, try to reduce your intake. That will help alleviate any imbalance that could develop. Get creative and try new foods from the list for your constitution. Regularly introduce new foods and try new recipes so that you have variety and an abundance of dishes to enjoy.

Favor cooked foods over raw. Steamed, lightly sautéed, baked, and grilled foods are good to include in the diet. Cooked foods are easier to digest than raw foods, and throughout this program, we want to increase the power of digestion, not diminish it. If you enjoy salads, opt to have your greens lightly steamed, rather than raw. If you like fruit smoothies, try cooking the fruit. To cook fruit, you can stew it in a pot with a little water and add some warming spices such as cinnamon and ginger. You can also bake fruit for a warm, delicious treat.

Food combining is important when it comes to balancing blood sugar. Make sure to include a good source of protein such as legumes, meat, nuts, or an egg with each meal. Protein will help reduce blood sugar spikes and satiate your hunger.

Include a handful of greens with your meals. If you are having scrambled eggs or an omelet in the morning, throw in a handful of spinach or arugula. For a quick, easy lunch, sauté a chicken breast with some bok choy and green beans and top with a tasty dressing. For dinner, try some wild rice with mung beans, fennel, and spinach. Leafy greens are easy to incorporate and do the body a lot of good when it comes to reducing inflammation and balancing blood sugar.

The key to success in this program is being prepared. There are lots of options available when it comes to meal preparation. We live in a society with just about every kitchen gadget you can imagine to prepare food. Find the tools you need to make your life easy, and invest in them. It's an investment in your health and commitment to this program.

Slow cookers (Crock-Pot® is one brand) are great for preparing delicious meals in advance. If you have a busy day ahead, prepare the meal in a slow cooker the night before so that it's ready in the morning. That way, you have a delicious bowl of food to put in a thermos and take for lunch. Slow cookers also work great for breakfast if your mornings are hectic. Try putting some amaranth, quinoa, and black rice in the slow cooker with a little coconut milk and cinnamon. The house will smell wonderful, and you will have a freshly prepared breakfast when you wake.

It's crucial to regularly grocery shop and have the foods that are recommended for your constitution accessible and available. Having these foods means you are less likely to indulge in foods that are not on the list. Before you begin the program, clear out your cupboards and refrigerator. Removing temptation will make it easier to follow your dietary plan. And if there is a slip up along the way, be kind to yourself and don't give up. We all make mistakes. If you find yourself in a situation with limited dietary options, try to choose something that is in alignment with and closely resembles foods from your plan. Avoid fried, sugary, or refined foods. Aim for wholesome, close-to-nature foods. The closer a food is to its natural state, the better it will be for you.

During the 12-week program, try to eat at home where you can prepare your own meals. When you prepare your own meals, you know the quality of the ingredients. When you create a meal at home, you infuse love and healing intention into it. Do you ever wonder why the meals prepared by your mother or grandmother always tasted so good? Someone else can make the exact meal with the exact same ingredients, and it just doesn't taste as good. According to Ayurvedic philosophy, the person who prepares the meal infuses it with loving energy. That doesn't happen when you eat at a restaurant! I understand that there may be an occasion when you will want to go out to eat, so prepare in advance. Look up the restaurant and find their menu online. Choose a dish that includes foods from your list, and ask the server to omit foods that are not on your list. For example, if you go to an Italian restaurant, order a dish that has chicken for the protein and a tomato sauce. If the dish has pasta, ask if they can double the vegetables and omit the noodles. You may have to get creative—that's why it's a good idea to look up the menu in advance.

It's important to eat three meals per day at regular mealtimes and avoid snacking. Eating at regular mealtimes will help balance the digestive fire, so that you are able to metabolize foods properly, with less metabolic waste. The digestive fire is strongest from 10 a.m. to 2 p.m., so consume the majority of your daily calories during those hours. Your body will have an easier time breaking down difficult-to-digest foods. If you consume meats, try to have them at lunch. This is different from the American tradition of having a big dinner in the evening, so do your best to get family members on board. Change is much easier when you have group support!

Mindful Eating Awareness

How, when, and where we eat are just as important as what we eat. Eating in a calm, relaxed state allows the body to rest, digest, and assimilate, letting food be medicine rather than a toxic burden on the body.

Mindful Eating Tips

- If you are not hungry in the morning, awaken with a thick coating on your tongue, or can still taste last night's dinner, forgo breakfast and allow your body more time to digest.
- Set an intention when you sit down for a meal. Allow yourself to become centered and be thankful for the food and the cook who prepared it.
- Eat in a peaceful and joyful place, where you feel happy and content.
- Eat the proper amount. Stop eating when you are about 50 percent full. This will allow enough room in your belly for optimal digestion.
- Eat three meals a day and reduce snacking.
- Eat at specific, regular times to improve digestive functioning.
- Eat warm or hot cooked foods; they are easier to digest than cold, raw foods.
- Reduce the chatter when you eat. Talking allows more air to enter the stomach, which can cause bloating and gas.
- Do not drink cold beverages with meals; it diminishes the digestive fire. If you are thirsty, sip on some warm water.
- Do not eat too fast or too slow. Try to consume meals within 30 minutes.
- Make lunch your biggest meal of the day. Digestion is strongest during the day. Try to finish lunch by 2 p.m.
- Eat every bite with mindfulness and enjoy the flavors.

- Eat only after the previous meal is digested (about 4 hours), and there is no coating on the tongue or taste of the previous meal in your mouth.
- Thoroughly chew every bite until it is liquid. Chewing is the first stage of digestion and will help with assimilation down the line.
- Finish dinner by 7 p.m. and avoid late night snacking, which forces your body to digest food when it needs to reserve energy for nightly detoxification.
- Eat with the seasons and according to your constitution. This helps promote healthy flora in the gut.
- Avoid distractions such as reading or watching TV while you are eating.
- Use culinary herbs and spices to upgrade the medicinal value of your meals. Cumin, coriander, turmeric, fennel, ginger, fenugreek, and cinnamon are all good choices.

Establishing a Daily Routine

Having a daily routine (or *dinacharya*) helps keep vata, pitta, and kapha in balance. The recommended daily routine varies depending on your constitution and the imbalance you are working to correct. The season, location, stage of life, and current condition are all factors to consider when developing a daily routine.

Our bodies love consistency, and we receive tremendous benefits from following a daily schedule. For example, making your main meal at lunchtime and eating a light dinner improves your digestion. Exercising and planning your day early in the morning increase mindfulness and productivity. Following a daily routine is like swimming with the current, whereas not following a routine is like swimming against the current. Daily routine helps regulate the flow of hormones, sleep/wake cycles, digestion, and assimilation. When we follow these cycles, we digest foods with less trouble, sleep better at night, and wake feeling less stiff. We feel well-rested in the morning and have more energy to do our morning exercise, which helps increase endorphins and other hormones that allow us to feel happy and peaceful throughout the day. Doesn't that sound great?

Walking After Meals

I recommend walking after meals for all constitutions with type 2 diabetes. The time spent walking varies depending on your constitution. Vata people require less, and kapha people need a little more. Walking is probably the easiest and most convenient exercise activity, and walking after meals reduces blood sugar.

Walking is a weight-bearing exercise with cardiovascular benefits. Following a regular walking routine reduces the risk of stroke and high blood pressure. Walking also creates a positive state of mind and reduces depression, anxiety, and tension.

When starting a walking routine, it's important to begin slowly to reduce the risk of injury. Muscles, joints, and ligaments need to be conditioned to prevent common injuries that can occur to the hamstrings, knees, and feet. By starting slowly, you can learn to read your body and comfort level. I recommend proper assessment by a professional trainer prior to starting the exercise program.

Improper surfaces or shoes, muscle weakness, inflexibility, and foot and alignment problems can lead to injuries if not dealt with properly. Finding the proper surface to walk on is important. Walking on a softer, level surface is ideal. A running track made of synthetic material absorbs more shock than concrete, making it easier on the knees and back.

A good pair of shoes is a necessity for walking. Proper footwear allows the feet to navigate various terrains in comfort. The foot moves naturally with a heel-to-toe rolling motion when wearing specially designed walking shoes. An athletic-footwear specialist can measure your feet and suggest the proper shoe to maximize your walking experience. Use clean, comfortable, athletic socks to keep the feet dry and free of blisters.

Your walking stride should feel natural and not overextended. If the stride is too long, the hamstrings will tend to tighten up, and knees and other joints may become sore. Always warm up by starting your walk at a slow pace for a couple of minutes, and increase speed from there.

Monitoring Your Intensity Level

1) **Speaking:** You should be able to say two to three sentences without gasping for breath while walking and working out.

2) **Capacity:** On a scale of 1 to 10, if sitting at rest is 0 and fully exerting yourself is 10, aim for a 5 when walking.

Determining Your Maximum Heart Rate

Determining your maximum heart rate (MHR) is beneficial when working out because it helps you stay in your ideal zone. This can help prevent injuries and reduce stress-hormone production. It helps you know when to pick up the pace and when to slow down. While walking, you can take a brief break to check your heart rate. The MHR for men is 220 minus age, and for women it is 226 minus age. For example, a 50-year-old man has an MHR of 170: 220–50 = 170. A 50-year-old man should therefore try to keep his heart rate under 170 beats per minute.

To check your heart rate, put your finger on your pulse. On the inside of your wrist, you will find your radial artery, and on either side of your windpipe is your carotid artery. You can take your pulse in either location. Have a timer or watch handy, and for 15 seconds count the number of pulses you feel, and then multiply that number by 4 to determine your heart rate per minute.

As you approach the end of your walk, allow a cool-down period for the tendons to loosen and relax. It isn't completely necessary to stretch before walking, but if you want to, stretch the calves, hamstrings, quads, buttocks, hip flexors, and groin for 20 to 30 seconds each.

Preventing Injuries

Exercise causes muscle growth. It is a natural process that occurs when muscles produce tiny tears that mend, grow, and become stronger. As this process happens, you can expect some slight stiffness or soreness the day following a good workout. Make sure you're relatively pain free before your next exercise session.

If you experience ongoing discomfort, you may have an injury. Foot or body structure may be the reason. Some people are overpronators, and others are supinators when they walk. The feet and ankles of overpronators naturally roll inward from the outside edge of the heel in toward the big toes instead of rolling straight along the bottom from heel to toe. Supinators have the opposite issue, as the feet roll outward. Various leg and knee injuries can result from either of these tendencies. Flat feet are another common characteristic that can cause discomfort. Custom insoles known as orthotics can correct foot problems. These insoles prevent motions that can lead to injuries. Overpronators or those with significant leg length differences often benefit from orthotics.

Various structural and muscular imbalances can adversely affect the knees. Walkers and weightlifters may experience knee problems. Women are more susceptible to knee problems than men are because they have wider hips, which affects the angle of the knee. If you have knee issues, it's important to focus on flexibility, strength, and stability to promote knee health and stay balanced. The knees need to be able to handle the workload placed on them. Strong, healthy, and flexible muscles protect the knees. Building muscles in the lower body will therefore support and stabilize the knees. A knee brace can also provide stability while exercising.

Most exercise injuries heal if they're dealt with quickly and efficiently. The RICE formula is effective for treating inflammation, pain, and swelling. RICE is an acronym for *rest, ice, compress,* and *elevate.*

RICE

REST: Continuing to walk with an injury will tend to make it worse, so discontinue exercise and rest.

ICE: Apply ice or a cold compress wrapped in a towel for the first 48 to 72 hours after the injury, for 15 minutes every 2 hours.

COMPRESS: Apply pressure to the area for the first couple of hours to decrease swelling. Wrap an elastic bandage around the area when you are up and moving around. Don't wear the bandage when elevating the injured area or when you go to bed.

ELEVATE: Keep the injured area elevated above your heart to decrease swelling and blood flow.

Dehydration can make you more prone to injury, so be sure to drink plenty of water. Half your body weight in ounces is the ideal daily amount; however, you may need more if you live in a hot climate or are walking great distances.

Discovering Your Constitution

It is essential to verify your constitution before beginning this program. Discovering your true nature will help determine the correct herbal formulations, amount of weekly exercise, and relaxation, sleep, and lifestyle recommendations for your constitution.

The program you follow in this book will vary depending on your constitution. Ayurveda offers personalized nutritional, lifestyle, and herbal guidelines to assist each person in harmonizing their constitution to bring them back into balance. In Ayurveda, two individuals with the same disease may receive very different treatment plans. For example, someone who is kapha-dominant may have to exercise more and sleep less than someone who is vata-dominant. Kapha people have more earth and water elements in their constitution, which contribute to heavy and slow qualities. They therefore need to bring more movement into the body. A person who is vata in nature has more air and ether, which creates a "windy" environment in their body and mind. It is essential for them to help calm and ground that energy. A vata person may require more sleep and relaxation therapies to balance their constitution. Pitta people have more heat and fire in their constitution, so they may benefit from a cooling, calming diet and stress reduction.

Ayurveda uses a system of health history, physical examination, observation, and pulse reading to determine a person's true nature and how they have deviated from their true nature to their current condition. In Ayurveda, we use three main diagnostic techniques: inspection, palpitation, and questioning. The practitioner observes the tongue, nails, and lips, as well as each of the body's nine "doors" (eyes [2], ears [2], nostrils [2], mouth, genitalia, and anus), along with their secretions. We examine secretions through questioning. We're not going to ask you to bring a stool sample in, but we're going to ask you a few questions about your bowel movements. The practitioner may listen to your breathing, look in your eyes, inspect your tongue, observe body language, and take your pulse to reveal strengths and weaknesses.

The Ayurvedic practitioner will take a detailed history to learn likes and dislikes, as well as past, present, and future health concerns. Through a 10-step process, traditionally called the tenfold examination, the Ayurvedic practitioner determines a person's constitution, discovers where imbalances lie, and assesses the quality of the physical tissues and bodily proportions. The practitioner also checks the client's mental strength and adaptability to stress, evaluates their digestive power, judges their exercise endurance, and determines their rate of aging.

A consultation with a certified Ayurvedic practitioner is the ideal way to determine your constitution. If you are not able to schedule an appointment with a practitioner, use the quiz below to help you determine your constitution. Please carefully read and complete the "Ayurveda Constitution Quiz" below. Answer the questions according to how you have experienced these mental qualities, behaviors, emotions, and physical characteristics for the majority of your life. If you feel like there are a couple of descriptions that represent you, check both. While it is difficult to determine your actual constitution without an examination, this will give you a good idea.

After you have determined your constitution, continue to the vata, pitta, or kapha program for balancing type 2 diabetes. Each program has variations that are specific to that constitution, and you should follow the program recommendations for your constitution.

AYURVEDA CONSTITUTION QUIZ

Instructions:

1. *Read across the page from left to right.*
2. *Each question has three columns. Check the boxes next to the options that best describe how you have behaved, felt, acted, or looked for the majority of your life.*
3. *If you feel that more than one of the descriptions apply to you, check all of those that accurately describe you.*
4. *After finishing the questionnaire, add up the number of items you checked in each of the columns. These numbers go in the totals row at the bottom of the quiz.*
5. *The column with the most checked items indicates your constitution.*

COLUMN 1	COLUMN 2	COLUMN 3
Hair:		
☐ Kinky, dry	☐ Thinning, light, premature grey	☐ Thick, oily
Nails:		
☐ Brittle, dry	☐ Pink, soft	☐ Strong, broad
Skin texture:		
☐ Dry, rough	☐ Soft, oily, warm	☐ Clammy, moist, cool
Body temperature:		
☐ Cold hands or feet	☐ Warm, runs hot	☐ Cool, clammy
Complexion:		
☐ Darker, tans easily	☐ Pink, freckles, burns quickly	☐ Pale, white
Veins:		
☐ Very prominent	☐ Fairly prominent	☐ Well covered
Eyes:		
☐ Small, unsteady	☐ Medium, sensitive to light	☐ Large, full lashes
Whites of eyes:		
☐ Dull	☐ Yellow or red	☐ Glossy white

Nose:

☐ Irregular, uneven   ☐ Sharp, pointed   ☐ Round, button

Lips:

☐ Thin, dry   ☐ Medium   ☐ Full, smooth

Cheeks:

☐ Wrinkled, sunken   ☐ Smooth, flat   ☐ Plump, round

Joints:

☐ Dry, cracking   ☐ Moderate, inflamed   ☐ Large, swollen

Weight as a child:

☐ Thin, hard to gain   ☐ Medium   ☐ Heavy, gained weight
  weight   easily

Elimination:

☐ Dry, hard, constipated   ☐ Many daily, loose   ☐ Large, regular

Indigestion:

☐ Gas, bloating   ☐ Heartburn, acidity,   ☐ Sluggishness, heaviness
                             nausea

Food sensitivities:

☐ Nightshades, dried fruits ☐ Citrus, acidic or spicy ☐ Dairy, wheat
                               foods

Tongue:

☐ Dry, cracked   ☐ Yellow central coating, ☐ White coating all over
                             red edges

Teeth:

☐ Irregular, crooked   ☐ Small to medium   ☐ Full, large, white

Gums:

☐ Receding   ☐ Sensitive, bleeding   ☐ Build tartar easily

Mouth:

☐ Dry   ☐ Sour taste   ☐ Excessive saliva

Muscle tone:

☐ Lean, ropy muscles   ☐ Loose, soft
☐ Good definition

Body frame:

☐ Thin, slim, or long   ☐ Medium frame   ☐ Large frame, fleshy

Urine:

☐ Scanty   ☐ Dark yellow, bloody, acidic   ☐ Cloudy, stringy, thick

Energy level:

☐ Fluctuates   ☐ Stable   ☐ Low

Appetite:

☐ Irregular, variable   ☐ Sharp, needs regular meals   ☐ Can easily miss meals

Snacking:

☐ When anxious, lonely   ☐ While concentrating   ☐ When depressed, sad

Mental activity:

☐ Active, busy   ☐ Focused, sharp   ☐ Calm mind

Memory recall:

☐ Short-term best   ☐ Good general memory   ☐ Long-term recall best

Attention span:

☐ Short attention span   ☐ Good   ☐ Tires easily

Dreams:

☐ Fearful, flying, running   ☐ Angry, violent, finances   ☐ Water, sweet, romance

Sleep:

☐ Insomnia, light   ☐ Difficulty falling asleep   ☐ Sound, heavy, difficult to wake

Routine:

☐ Does not like to follow   ☐ Prefers to create own   ☐ Does better if someone else creates

Decision-making:

☐ Indecisive   ☐ Focused, quick decisions   ☐ Slow and thoughtful

Friendships:

☐ Many short-term   ☐ Few, long-lasting friendships

☐ Loner, friends at work

Dating history:

☐ Many casual   ☐ Intense, passionate   ☐ Long and deep

Activity level:

☐ Constantly moving   ☐ Moderately active   ☐ Prefers to relax

Best working environment:

☐ While supervised   ☐ Needs to be the leader   ☐ In groups

Weather:

☐ Aversion to cold   ☐ Aversion to heat   ☐ Aversion to rain, humidity

Finances:

☐ Spends quickly   ☐ Saves, but big spender   ☐ Saves, accumulates

Competition:

☐ Don't like pressure   ☐ Driven competitor   ☐ Passive

Speech:

☐ Fast, may skip words   ☐ Sharp, clear cut   ☐ Slow, sweet

Voice:

☐ Hoarse, dry   ☐ Distinct pitch   ☐ Low, melodious pitch

Moods and emotions:

☐ Change quickly   ☐ Easily irritated   ☐ Steady, stable, calm

Reaction to stress:

☐ Fear   ☐ Anger   ☐ Indifference

Emotionally sensitive to:

☐ Own feelings   ☐ Not sensitive   ☐ Others' feelings

Sexual activity:

☐ Tires easily   ☐ Strong desire   ☐ Slow to arouse

Expressions of affection:

☐ With words   ☐ With gifts   ☐ With touch, affection

Trauma causes:

☐ Anxiety   ☐ Denial   ☐ Depression

Total Column #1: VATA	Total Column #2: PITTA	Total Column #3: KAPHA

Once you have completed the quiz, add up the number of items you checked in each column to find the total. The column with the highest total indicates your constitution. If you have two columns that are equal or very close, it indicates that you are dual constitution. Many people will have a secondary dosha that is almost equal to their primary dosha. If this occurs, retake the test and answer the questions according to how you currently feel, act, behave, and look. You may find some of your answers will change. This will indicate the dosha that is out of balance. Next proceed to the chapter for the 8-week constitution and elimination diet for your constitution:

The vata program starts on page 71 (Chapter 6).

The pitta program begins on page 100 (Chapter 7).

The kapha program starts on page 127 (Chapter 8).

The 12-Week Program: 8-Week Constitution and Elimination Diet for Vata

Your goal for the first 8 weeks of the program is to eat foods that help ground and balance vata without being overly heavy, sweet, or salty. Vata people tend to have variable digestion. It's essential to keep mealtimes regular; this will help regulate the digestive secretions and hormones that promote balanced digestion. It's critical to eat three meals per day at the same time each day and to avoid snacking. Eating at regular mealtimes will help balance the digestive fire so that you can metabolize foods properly and have less metabolic waste. The digestive fire is robust during the hours of 10 a.m. to 2 p.m., so consume the majority of your daily calories during those hours. Your body will have an easier time breaking down challenging-to-digest foods. If you consume meat, try to have it at lunch. Transition away from a big dinner and opt for a larger lunch.

Try to eat in a relaxed environment. When it's time to eat, sit down and enjoy your meal. Don't eat on the go. Mindfully chew your food, enjoy the flavors in each bite, and take your time. In Ayurveda, it is believed that digestion starts in the mouth. When we experience tastes, this stimulates the other digestive organs. Sour promotes salivation, stimulates secretions in the stomach, and improves the digestive process. Sour is the taste that is most beneficial for a vata person with high blood sugar. It is warming, so it balances the cold nature of vata. It is also grounding, so it helps counterbalance the irregular fluctuations a vata person can have with their blood sugar. Sour is cleansing and refreshing; it encourages the elimination of waste and alleviates constipation. Sour is excellent for removing air from the body; it dispels gas and reduces bloating. Sour increases the digestive fire by stimulating acidic secretions in the stomach. All these actions are beneficial for strengthening the digestive fire and improving vata digestion and metabolism. Beyond the digestive process, sour enhances circulation, benefiting the cardiovascular system, along with sensory and neurological functioning.

The sour taste is in fermented and acidic foods. Citrus fruits and fermented products have a therapeutic heating effect, beneficial for vata. However, it is essential to avoid fermented milk products, wine, and alcohol during the 12-week program. Examples of sour foods that are beneficial for a vata person with type 2 diabetes include lemons, limes, raspberries, vinegar, and tamarind. To include more lemon in your diet, try squeezing a fresh lemon on a prepared meal. Incorporate apple cider vinegar into soups, sauces, and stews to add a little sour zing. Tamarind is a unique sour fruit that is used as a condiment in Indian and Asian cuisine. It helps balance heavy foods and makes them easier to digest. I like to mix a little tamarind on seeds and nuts. A little goes a long way, so use discretion with tamarind.

Here is a list of low-glycemic foods that benefit the vata constitution. Please include these foods in your 8-week constitution and elimination diet.

Vata Food Lists

Fruits to enjoy: cooked apples, apple sauce, avocado, blackberries, blueberries, cherries, coconut, elderberries, goose berries, goji berries, grapefruit, grapes, jackfruit (ripe), kiwi, lemons, limes, oranges, pineapple, plums, prunes, raspberries, rhubarb, strawberries

Fruits to avoid: raw apples, cranberries, dried dates and most other dried fruits, pears, persimmons, watermelon

Vegetables to enjoy (vegetables should be cooked): asparagus, beets, bok choy, carrots, cucumber, daikon radish, fennel, garlic, green beans, mild green chilis, jackfruit (unripe), leafy greens, leeks, lettuce, mustard greens, okra, black olives, onion, peas, parsnip, radishes, rutabaga, spaghetti squash, spinach, sprouts, summer squash, taro root, turnip greens, watercress, zucchini, kelp, seaweed, scallions

Vegetables to enjoy in moderation: artichoke, cabbage, corn, eggplant, tomatoes

Vegetables to avoid (generally frozen, dried, or raw): bell peppers, broccoli, Brussels sprouts, burdock root, cauliflower, celery, green olives, horseradish, hot peppers, mushrooms, potatoes, turnips, winter squash, wheatgrass

Grains to enjoy: amaranth, barley, black rice, brown rice, steel cut oats, quinoa, wild rice

Grains to avoid: buckwheat, pre-packaged cereals, couscous, millet, white rice, rye, spelt, tapioca, wheat

Legumes to enjoy: red lentils, mung beans, mung dal, green peas, tempeh

Legumes to avoid: azuki beans, black beans, black-eyed peas, black lentils, chickpeas (garbanzo beans), kidney beans, brown lentils, lima beans, navy beans, pigeon peas, pinto beans, soybeans, split peas, white beans

Dairy to enjoy: ghee

Avoid all other dairy.

Meats and eggs to enjoy: chicken (white meat), turkey (white meat), eggs

Meats to avoid: beef, duck, fish, lamb, pork, shellfish, venison

Condiments to enjoy: black pepper, ketchup, kimchi, mustard, pickles, sauerkraut, soy sauce, tamari, apple cider vinegar, liquid amino acids, tahini

Condiments to avoid: horseradish

Nuts to enjoy (in moderation): almonds, brazil nuts, cashews, coconut, filberts/hazelnuts, macadamia, peanuts, pecans, pine nuts, pistachios, walnuts

No nuts to avoid!

Seeds to enjoy: chia, flax, pumpkin, sesame, sunflower

Seeds to avoid: popcorn

Oils to enjoy (organic, cold-pressed): sesame, ghee, olive, avocado, almond

No oils to avoid!

Beverages to enjoy: coconut milk, unsweetened coconut water, warm almond milk, unsweetened soft cider, decaffeinated unsweetened herbal chai tea, unsweetened grapefruit juice, unsweetened lemonade, miso broth, unsweetened warm soy milk

Beverages to avoid: alcohol, black tea, green tea, iced tea, coffee, other caffeinated beverages, carbonated drinks, chocolate milk, dairy drinks, cranberry juice, icy drinks, pear juice, cold soy milk, tomato juice, V8® juice

---

Herbs to enjoy: basil, catnip, chamomile, chicory, cilantro, elderflower, eucalyptus, fenugreek, ginger (fresh), juniper berry, kukicha, lavender, lemongrass, licorice, marshmallow, oat straw, oregano, parsley, peppermint, raspberry, rosehips, rosemary, saffron, sage, sarsaparilla, sassafras, spearmint, strawberry leaf, thyme, wintergreen

Herbs to avoid: aloe vera, corn silk, dandelion, ginseng, hibiscus, jasmine, lemon balm, nettle, passionflower, red clover, yarrow, yerba mate

---

Sweeteners to enjoy (in small amounts): apple sauce, honey, molasses

Sweeteners to avoid: barley malt, fruit juice concentrates, maple syrup, white and brown sugar

---

Spices to enjoy: All spices are good!

Recipes for Vata

BASIC RECIPES

GINGER LEMONADE

This refreshing drink contains citrus, which strengthens the digestive fire, and ginger to clear metabolic waste from the lymph and blood.

Makes: Four 8-ounce glasses

Ingredients:

- 4 cups water
- Juice of 1 lemon
- Juice of ½ lime
- 1 teaspoon grated fresh ginger

Instructions:

Combine water, lemon juice, lime juice, and ginger in a blender. Process on high for 30 seconds.

ARTICHOKE TAHINI

Artichoke tahini is a great addition to your pantry since it can be used as a dip, a dressing, and a sauce.

Makes: 4 servings

Ingredients:

- 1 can (14 ounces) artichoke hearts, drained
- ¼ cup tahini
- ¼ cup chopped fresh herbs, such as rosemary, cilantro, basil, and/or parsley
- 1 head roasted garlic (see page 76)
- 2 tablespoons freshly squeezed lemon or lime juice
- ¼ to ½ cup extra-virgin olive oil

Instructions:

1. Combine the artichoke hearts, tahini, herbs, and garlic in the bowl of a food processor. Process for 20 seconds. With the motor running, add lemon juice and slowly pour ¼ cup of the oil through the funnel in the lid.
2. Scrape down the sides and check the consistency. With the motor running, slowly add more oil through the funnel to gradually thin the mixture to the desired consistency: thick if you want to use it as a spread or dip, thinner for a sauce or dressing.

PESTO

Pine nuts, a common ingredient in pesto, satiate the body and provide nourishment.

If you are unable to use pine nuts, substitute any nut on the vata food list.

Makes: 2 cups

Ingredients:

- ¼ cup pine nuts
- 2 cups lightly packed fresh basil
- Juice of ½ lemon
- ½ teaspoon ground fenugreek
- ¼ teaspoon ground turmeric
- about 1 cup extra-virgin olive oil

Instructions:

Coarsely chop the nuts in a food processor. Add basil and sprinkle lemon juice, fenugreek, and turmeric on top. With the motor running, slowly add half of the oil through the funnel in the lid and process for about 1 minute, stopping to scrape down the sides of the bowl, and check the consistency of the pesto. For a smoother, thinner consistency, slowly add the remaining oil.

ROASTED GARLIC

Garlic has cleansing anti-viral, antimicrobial, and anti-fungal actions. Individual cloves of garlic grow around the stem in a cluster, and each cluster of cloves is called a "head." This recipe calls for four whole clusters or heads of garlic.

Makes: about ½ cup roasted garlic

Ingredients:

- 4 heads garlic
- 1 tablespoon extra-virgin olive oil

Instructions:

1. Preheat oven to 400° F and line a rimmed baking sheet with parchment paper.
2. Scrape off any roots and slice ¼ inch off the top of each head. Rub between your palms to remove loose leaves. Place each head, cut side up, on the prepared baking sheet. Drizzle oil over the tops.
3. Bake in preheated oven for 1 hour or until flesh is golden and very soft. Store roasted garlic in the heads and squeeze flesh out when needed, or cool the heads and squeeze the soft flesh out of the skin into a small bowl. Store for 1 to 2 weeks in an airtight container in the refrigerator.

VATA BREAKFAST

BARLEY AND SPINACH SCRAMBLE

Egg whites are a good source of protein, and the yolks are warming and nourish vata. The combination of eggs, greens, and barley make a high-fiber and high-protein breakfast, perfect for vata.

Makes: 2 servings

Ingredients:

- 1 tablespoon extra-virgin sesame oil or ghee (see page 164)
- ¼ onion, chopped (about ¼ cup)
- 2 cups packed baby spinach or roughly chopped mature spinach
- ½ cup cooked barley (see page 21)
- 2 eggs, beaten

Instructions:

1. Heat oil in a skillet over medium-high heat. Add onion and cook, stirring frequently for 5 minutes or until soft and translucent. Add spinach and cook, stirring constantly for 1 minute, or until spinach is wilted.
2. Stir in the barley. Pour eggs over and cook, stirring constantly for 3 to 4 minutes, or until the eggs are cooked and the barley is warmed through.

WARM BARLEY BREAKFAST BOWL

Hearty and warming, this bowl starts you off on a solid footing for balancing blood-sugar levels while providing lots of energy for the morning. Make double the amount and have a bowl for lunch as well.

Makes: 1 serving

Ingredients:

- 1 tablespoon ghee, divided
- 1 cup cooked barley (see page 21)
- 2 cups packed baby spinach or roughly chopped mature spinach
- 1 hardboiled egg, sliced
- 2 tablespoons raw sunflower seeds
- 1 teaspoon raw sesame seeds

Instructions:

1. Heat half of the ghee in a skillet over medium-low heat. Add barley and stir constantly for about 2 minutes or until warmed through.
2. Spoon the barley into a cereal bowl. Add the remaining ghee and the spinach to the skillet. Cover, reduce heat to low, and cook for 1 minute or until the spinach is wilted. Add to the barley in the bowl. Arrange egg around spinach, and sprinkle sunflower and sesame seeds on top.

Note: If you have just cooked the barley, you don't need to reheat it, so skip step 1 and use the full quantity of ghee in step 2.

CHIA SEED PUDDING

Chia seed pudding is nourishing and delicious. Chia seeds are unique because they absorb water and become gelatinous, which promotes healthy elimination. This recipe also makes a great dessert.

Makes: 2 servings

Ingredients:

- 2 cups water
- ¼ fresh vanilla bean
- 2 tablespoons extra-virgin coconut oil
- ¼ teaspoon ground cinnamon
- ⅛ teaspoon ground cardamom
- ⅛ teaspoon ground nutmeg
- ½ cup chia seeds
- 5 raw almonds, coarsely chopped

Instructions:

1. Pour water into a blender. Split the vanilla bean and scrape the tiny seeds into the water. Add coconut oil, cinnamon, cardamom, and nutmeg. Cover and blend on high for 1 minute or until well mixed. Pour into a bowl and stir in the chia seeds. Cover and set aside for 30 minutes.
2. Spoon into two bowls. Divide chopped almonds in half and sprinkle over each bowl.

GREEN EGG FRITTATA

Make this breakfast dish seasonal by using asparagus in the spring, green beans in the summer, and chopped leafy greens such as spinach, Swiss chard, or finely chopped kale in the fall and winter.

Makes: 1 or 2 servings

Ingredients:

- 1 tablespoon ghee (see page 164)
- ¼ onion, chopped (about ¼ cup)
- 1 cup chopped fresh asparagus (see headnote, above)
- 3 eggs, lightly beaten

Instructions:

1. Melt ghee in a skillet over medium-high heat. Stir in onion and asparagus and cook, stirring frequently, for 5 minutes or until onions are soft and translucent and asparagus is crisp-tender.
2. Pour eggs over and lower heat to medium-low. Cook, stirring frequently, for about 2 minutes or until the eggs are cooked through.

OVERNIGHT OAT-APPLE BOWL

Oats are a good source of fiber and antioxidants. If purchased from a mill that does not process wheat, they are gluten-free. Look for large-flake, steel-cut oats if possible. Avoid instant oats. Make this your own by replacing the apple with other seasonal, vata-friendly fruit, adding shredded coconut or nuts, or swapping ginger for the cinnamon.

Makes: 1 serving

Ingredients:

- ½ cup almond milk (plus more for serving)
- ½ cup steel-cut oats
- 1 tablespoon chia seeds
- ¼ teaspoon ground cinnamon or ginger
- 1 apple, chopped
- 1 tablespoon chopped raw almonds or unsweetened coconut

Instructions:

1. The night before, combine milk, oats, chia seeds, and cinnamon in a bowl. Cover and set in the refrigerator overnight.
2. In the morning, remove from refrigerator and transfer to a small, lightly oiled saucepan. Stir in the chopped apple and warm over medium heat, stirring constantly, for 1 minute or until warmed through. Serve hot or warm with almonds sprinkled on top.

Alternative method—use a double boiler: To save a step and make this oil-free, combine milk, oats, chia seeds, and cinnamon in the top of a double boiler. Cover and refrigerate. In the morning, bring an inch of water in the bottom of the double boiler to a boil. Fit the top boiler over the bottom, cover, and heat, stirring frequently for 1 minute or until warmed through. If you do not have a double boiler, a heatproof bowl that fits over a saucepan (but does not touch the bottom of the pan) will work just as well.

VATA LUNCH

MUNG BEAN AND BARLEY STEW

Hing, also known as asafetida, is used as a culinary herb in Ayurvedic cooking. Hing expels gas and reduces bloating. Include a little hing as you soak your beans to improve digestion. Serve with sautéed or steamed veggies.

Makes: 4 servings

Ingredients:

- 2 cups dried mung beans, well rinsed
- Pinch of hing/asafetida
- 1 tablespoon ghee (see page 164) or extra-virgin sunflower oil
- 1 onion, chopped

- 3 cloves garlic, minced
- 2 tablespoons freshly grated ginger
- 1 teaspoon ground turmeric
- ½ cup hulled barley
- 4 cups packed baby spinach or roughly chopped mature spinach

Instructions:

1. The night before, cover beans with 6 cups of water in a large pot. Add hing and set aside to soak overnight.
2. The next day, drain and rinse the beans in a colander. Set aside.
3. Warm ghee in a large pot over medium heat. Add onion and cook, stirring frequently, for 4 minutes. Add garlic and ginger and cook, stirring frequently, for 2 to 3 minutes or until onion is soft and translucent.
4. Stir in turmeric and 3 cups of water. Increase heat to high and bring to a boil. Add barley. Reduce heat to low, cover, and simmer for 20 minutes. Check that there is at least ½ cup of water left; if not, add water and bring to a simmer. Stir in beans and continue to simmer for about 10 minutes or until the barley and beans are tender.
5. Remove from heat, cool, stir in spinach, and serve at room temperature.

CHICKEN TACO SALAD WITH AVOCADO DRESSING

Chicken is a low glycemic food and grounding for vata. This muscle-building recipe will help you feel nourished and energized.

Makes: 2 servings

Ingredients:

Chicken taco salad:
- 1 tablespoon ghee (see page 164) or extra-virgin sesame oil
- 1 boneless, skinless chicken breast, coarsely chopped
- 2 cups chopped kale
- about 1 cup vegetable broth or water

Avocado dressing:
- 1 avocado
- 1 cup coarsely chopped fresh cilantro
- 1 tablespoon freshly squeezed lemon juice
- ¼ teaspoon ground turmeric
- 1 tablespoon water

Instructions:

1. Heat ghee in a small skillet over medium-high heat. Add chicken and cook, stirring constantly, for 1 minute to brown. Add kale and enough broth to cover it and the chicken pieces. Cover, lower the heat to medium-low, and

simmer for 5 to 7 minutes or until the center of the chicken turns opaque and the internal temperature reaches 165° F.

2. Meanwhile, make the avocado dressing. Cut avocado in half, remove the seed, and scoop the flesh into a blender. Add cilantro, lemon juice, turmeric, and water and blend on high until smooth.
3. When the chicken is cooked, remove from heat and drain any excess liquid. Drizzle avocado dressing on top and toss.

CHICKEN WITH BOK CHOY

Bok choy is a superfood. It is an excellent source of vitamins A, C, and K, and it contains over 70 antioxidants that help prevent inflammatory conditions related to type 2 diabetes. Cooking the chicken with the bones in infuses the broth with minerals from them.

Makes: 4 to 6 servings

Ingredients:

- ½ chicken, bone in
- 1 can (14 ounces) coconut milk
- 2 ½ cups water
- 1 cup wild rice
- 1 bunch bok choy, coarsely chopped
- 1 tablespoon chopped or ground dried kelp
- 1 tablespoon apple cider vinegar
- 1 teaspoon ground fenugreek
- 1 teaspoon ground turmeric

Instructions:

1. Cut chicken into two or three pieces, leaving the bones in. Remove and discard the skin.
2. Combine coconut milk and water in a large slow cooker. Stir in rice, bok choy, kelp, vinegar, fenugreek, and turmeric. Add the chicken, pushing it down into the liquid.
3. Set temperature to low, cover, and cook for 4 hours. Check the internal temperature of the chicken breast. It should read 165° F. If not, set the temperature to high, cover, and cook for an hour or until the temperature reaches 165° F.
4. Lift out the chicken and cool slightly. Remove the skin and bones, cut the meat into small pieces, and return them to the liquid before serving.

THAI RED CURRY CHICKEN

Red curry has a medium heat—warmer than yellow and cooler than green.

Substitute any curry for more or less spice, and try with a variety of vegetables on the vata food list.

Makes: 6 servings

Ingredients:

- 1 can (14 ounces) coconut milk
- 2 ½ cups water
- 2 tablespoons Thai red curry paste or powder
- ½ chicken, bone-in, cut into 3 or 4 pieces, skin removed
- 1 small onion, chopped
- 1 cup chopped asparagus
- 1 cup chopped green beans
- 1 cup chopped carrot
- 1 cup wild rice

Instructions:

1. Combine milk, water, and curry paste in a slow cooker. Add chicken pieces, onion, asparagus, green beans, carrot, and rice and stir to combine.
2. Cover and set temperature to low. Cook for 6 hours or until the internal temperature of a larger chicken piece reaches 165° F.
3. Lift out the chicken and cool slightly. Remove skin and bones, cut the meat into small pieces, and return them to liquid before serving.

GREEN CHILI TURKEY BURGERS

Turkey helps the body relax, and the green chilis add flavor and heat to promote digestion. Rosemary clears toxins, and the lettuce provides a healthy, low-glycemic bun.

Makes: 4 burgers

Ingredients:

- 1 pound ground turkey
- 1 tablespoon finely chopped fresh green chili pepper
- 1 tablespoon chopped fresh rosemary or parsley
- about 1 tablespoon extra-virgin coconut oil
- 1 head Boston lettuce, leaves separated

Instructions:

1. Combine turkey, chili, and rosemary in a bowl. Lightly oil the palms of your hands, and mix well by hand. Form into four patties.
2. Heat the oil in a large skillet over medium heat. Cook the patties for about 3 to 4 minutes on each side or until golden brown and cooked through. Turkey is cooked when the internal temperature reaches 165° F. Serve each patty between two lettuce leaves.

QUINOA BOWL WITH LENTILS AND VEGETABLES

This makes a beautiful presentation when served in a glass salad bowl, but you can layer the ingredients directly into four or six individual bowls. Try different cooked, seasonal, vata-friendly vegetables every time you make it.

Makes: 4 to 6 servings

Ingredients:

- 2 cups water or vegetable stock
- 1 cup quinoa, well rinsed
- 3 tablespoons ghee (see page 164) or extra-virgin olive oil, divided
- 1 onion, chopped
- 2 cloves garlic, finely chopped
- ½ teaspoon ground chili pepper
- ¼ teaspoon ground coriander
- ¼ teaspoon ground cumin
- 1 cup fresh or frozen (defrosted) corn kernels
- 1 cup fresh or frozen (defrosted) 1-inch pieces green beans
- 1 cup chopped fresh or frozen (defrosted) kale or cabbage
- 2 avocados
- 2 tablespoons freshly squeezed lime juice
- 1 can (15 ounces) red lentils, rinsed and drained

Instructions:

1. Bring water to a boil in a saucepan over high heat. Stir in quinoa and reduce heat to medium-high to keep water gently boiling. Cook for 8 to 10 minutes or until tender. Set a fine-mesh strainer over the sink and drain. Transfer quinoa back to the empty pot, toss with 1 tablespoon of the ghee, and set aside.

2. Meanwhile, heat remaining ghee in a large skillet over medium-high heat. Add onion and cook, stirring occasionally for 5 minutes or until translucent. Stir in garlic, chili, coriander, and cumin. Add corn, green beans, and kale. Cook, stirring constantly, for 7 minutes (less if using frozen vegetables) or until vegetables are crisp-tender.

3. Peel and dice avocados. Toss with lime juice in a small bowl.

4. To assemble: Spoon quinoa into a large glass or wooden salad bowl. Scrape cooked vegetable mixture over quinoa. Spread lentils over vegetables and sprinkle avocados and juice on top.

MUNG BEAN AND COCONUT CURRY

Mung beans are a low-calorie, low-glycemic food. They are used in Ayurveda to reduce inflammation in the digestive system, balance blood sugar, and heal the body.

Makes: 4 servings

Ingredients:
- 2 cups dried mung beans, well rinsed
- Pinch of hing or asafetida (see headnote, page 79)
- 2 tablespoons ghee (see page 164) or extra-virgin sesame oil
- 9 cloves garlic, crushed
- 2 tablespoons curry powder
- 2 tablespoons freshly grated ginger
- 3 cups water
- 1 can (14 ounces) coconut milk
- 3 cups coarsely chopped kale
- 1 avocado
- Juice of 1 lime

Instructions:
1. The night before, cover beans with 6 cups of water in a large pot. Stir in hing and set aside to soak overnight.
2. The next day, drain beans in a colander and rinse well. Heat ghee in a large pot over medium-low heat. Add garlic and cook, stirring constantly, for 3 to 4 minutes or until browned, but watch carefully so that it doesn't burn.
3. Stir in curry powder and ginger and cook, stirring constantly, for 1 minute. Add the water and mung beans. Increase heat to high and bring the mixture to a boil. Cover, reduce heat to low, and simmer for 20 minutes, stirring the mixture once or twice. Test a few mung beans to make sure they are tender. If not, continue to simmer for 10 minutes or until the beans are tender.
4. Stir in the coconut milk and kale. Bring to a boil and then immediately turn off the heat. Peel and slice the avocado. Stir avocado and lime juice into beans and serve hot.

BARLEY POLENTA

In this recipe, the barley becomes crisp on the outside and creamy in the middle. You can serve this with roasted vegetables or vegetable spirals. You can also drizzle it with tahini or pesto (page 75) or add cooked chicken.

Makes: 4 servings

Ingredients:
- 1 cup hulled barley
- 2 cups water
- 1 tablespoon extra-virgin almond oil or sunflower oil

Instructions:

1. The night before, bring a saucepan of water to a boil over medium-high heat. Stir in barley, cover, and simmer for 40 minutes or until tender. Drain and rinse with cold water.
2. Tightly pack barley into a storage container, using a spoon to press it down. Pack the barley until it measures about 1 inch thick. Cover and chill in the refrigerator for 24 hours.
3. The next night, cut the brick of barley into 1-inch-wide slices.
4. Heat oil in a skillet over medium heat. Add barley sticks and cook for 3 to 5 minutes or until lightly browned. Flip and cook for 3 to 4 minutes or until sticks are lightly browned on the opposite side.

SPAGHETTI SQUASH WITH KALE AND GARLIC

Use spaghetti squash as you would pasta, accenting it with different sauces and a mixture of roasted carrots, onions, leafy greens, and/or summer squash. Add fresh basil and olive oil for a simple and filling yet light dinner.

Makes: 6 servings

Ingredients:

- 1 spaghetti squash
- 1 tablespoon extra-virgin olive oil
- 1 tablespoon ghee (see page 164)
- 2 cups chopped kale
- 1 cup chopped green cabbage
- 1 tablespoon minced garlic
- ½ teaspoon ground fenugreek
- ¼ teaspoon ground turmeric
- Pinch of black pepper

Instructions:

1. Preheat oven to 375° F. Line a rimmed baking sheet with parchment paper.
2. Cut squash in half lengthwise, scoop out seeds, and drizzle the cut sides with oil. Place cut side down on prepared baking sheet. Roast in preheated oven for 40 minutes or until the flesh is easy to shred.
3. Meanwhile, heat ghee in a large skillet over medium heat. Add kale and cabbage. Cook, stirring frequently, for 4 minutes. Add garlic, fenugreek, turmeric, and pepper and cook for 2 more minutes or until garlic is translucent.
4. Scoop cooked spaghetti squash into a serving bowl or platter. Scrape cooked kale mixture on top and serve hot.

RED LENTIL PASTA

Fresh, seasonal vegetables are best, but some canned vegetables such as tomatoes and legumes are convenient to use. When purchasing canned vegetables, look for BPA-free can linings and steer clear of added sugar, salt, and preservatives. Make this dish seasonal by using fresh asparagus in the spring instead of beans. If using asparagus, add it with the pasta in step 3.

Makes: 4 to 6 servings

Ingredients:

- 2 tablespoons extra-virgin coconut oil, divided
- 1 onion, chopped
- 1 pound ground turkey or chicken
- 1 can (28 ounces) diced tomatoes with their juices
- 1 cup chopped cauliflower
- 1 cup roughly chopped fresh green beans
- 1 cup water
- 1 cup red lentil penne pasta
- ½ cup fresh or frozen (thawed) green peas

Instructions:

1. Heat 1 tablespoon of the oil in a large pot over medium-high heat. Add onion and cook, stirring frequently, for 4 minutes. Add turkey and stir, breaking it up with a wooden spoon. Cook, stirring occasionally, for 10 minutes or until the meat shows no sign of pink.

2. Add the tomatoes and their juices and bring to a boil. Stir in cauliflower and beans. Cover and reduce heat to medium-low. Simmer, stirring occasionally, for 8 minutes.

3. Stir in water and pasta and bring to a boil over high heat. Cover, reduce heat to low, and cook for 9 minutes or until pasta is al dente and vegetables are crisp-tender. Stir in peas and heat through.

Sleep Optimization

The classic Ayurvedic text *Charaka Samhita* states that "sleep is one of the main pillars of health—happiness, misery, nourishment, emaciation, strength, weakness, virility, knowledge, ignorance, life, death—all these occur depending on proper or improper sleep."

Vata people may have the most insomnia and sleep-related issues. Due to their natural physiology, they have more movement in the body and mind, and it can be difficult for them to fall asleep and stay asleep. They spend many restless nights tossing and turning and waking frequently, and they do not feel well rested in the morning. Symptoms of insomnia include sleeplessness, difficulty falling asleep, difficulty maintaining sleep, and feeling lethargic throughout the day. Insomnia affects millions of people worldwide and is very common throughout the world due to the modern lifestyle. Around 30 to 40 percent of Americans experience insomnia. Insomnia is more likely to affect women and elderly adults. According to Ayurveda, as we age, we move into the vata stage of life, and this life transition contributes to difficulty sleeping.

Hectic lifestyles, late dinners, and stress are all contributing factors to insomnia. Research has shown that 50 percent of insomnia cases are due to a mental or emotional imbalance. I have included a daily relaxation practice for vata people. If you have difficulty falling asleep, I recommend practicing it before bed. The relaxation program will allow you to calm your mind and prepare your body for sleep.

Insomnia can become a serious contributing factor to many chronic diseases such as type 2 diabetes, hypertension, and depression. Insomnia promotes insulin resistance, which can result in diabetes. Weight gain is also a typical result of sleep loss. When we get less than 6 hours of sleep, the body produces a stress hormone called cortisol. Cortisol directs the body to go into fat-storage mode. Blood moves away from the organs and into the limbs. Cortisol shuts down digestion, decreasing nutrient absorption and halting the production of digestive enzymes and acids. We store fat rather than burn it.

Cortisol also causes carbohydrate cravings. The body craves simple sugars to use for immediate energy. The body has this same reaction to stress, whether the stress is mental or physical. Stress causes your respiratory rate, heart rate, and blood pressure to increase. In response to a stressful trigger, the body produces cortisol and prepares for physical action. Most of the stress we experience today is mental. Stress from work, lack of sleep, or a blood sugar crash—all these kinds of stress produce the same physical reaction, which is likely to occur more than 30 times throughout the day. When mental stress occurs and your muscles are not engaged, glucose uptake does not occur. Hyperglycemia is harmful for someone who is diabetic or overweight. Getting a good night's sleep and reducing stress are vital components in this program.

Ayurveda promotes removing the root cause to correct an imbalance. When addressing sleep issues, it is essential to look at your diet and lifestyle and remove critical factors that could contribute to difficulty sleeping.

Causes of Insomnia
- Overeating
- Undereating
- Spicy foods

- Exercising close to bedtime
- Uncomfortable bed
- Environment—too noisy, too light, too cold, or too hot
- Sleeping late
- Pain or injury
- Staying up late
- Jet lag
- Use of electronic screens at night
- Emotions—anger, greed, excitement, grief, stress
- Stimulants—caffeine, alcohol

If any of these diet or lifestyle factors are affecting your sleep, try to correct them. Remember that 50 percent of insomnia cases are due to mental and emotional issues, so if you are experiencing more stress than usual, practice your relaxation program before bed.

Recommendations for Getting a Good Night's Sleep
- Find a soft pillow and mattress.
- Drink a cup of almond milk with 1/8 tsp of freshly grated nutmeg before bed.
- Write a list of things that you plan to do tomorrow before you go to bed.
- Rub your feet with warm sesame oil and put on a pair of warm socks before bed.
- Go to bed before 10 p.m.
- Eat a vata-reducing diet, especially for dinner.
- Practice calm, deep belly-breathing exercises.
- Avoid napping.
- Make sure your bedroom is dark and quiet; no electronics in the bedroom.
- Enjoy a light dinner at least 2 hours before going to bed.
- Do not read the news or watch TV before bed or in bed.
- Put all electronics away 1 hour before bed.
- Practice your relaxation program before bed.

Vata Daily Schedule
Wake up: 5:30–6:00 a.m.
30-minute resistance training
Breakfast: 7:30–8:30 a.m.
10-minute walk

Lunch: 11:30–12:30 p.m.
10-minute walk
Dinner: 5:30–6:30 p.m.
10-minute walk
Relaxation practice
Go to sleep: 9:30–10:00 p.m.

Lifestyle Enhancement

Vatas tend to have more difficulty dealing with stress, so the lifestyle-enhancement program developed for vata emphasizes the importance of stress management. The relaxation exercises include slowing down the breath to relax the body.

Allow 30 minutes for your relaxation practice. It includes yoga poses, breathwork, and meditation. If you are new to these practices, don't be afraid to give them a try. The yoga poses are gentle and restorative. Yoga has been shown to improve sleep length and quality. The recommended breathwork is soothing, and you may notice an immediate effect. The meditation is a simple exercise that you can do on your own or with guided audio.

Include your relaxation practice as part of your daily routine. Aim for 30 minutes, but if you can't get 30 minutes in and can only do 10 minutes, please do it for 10 minutes. A little is better than nothing, and consistency is more beneficial than irregularity. Once you begin to explore your relaxation practice, you may find that you gravitate toward one activity over another. If that happens, feel free to alter the times spent in each activity.

I recommend setting a timer during your relaxation practice so that you can be fully present and enjoy your time.

30-Minute Daily Relaxation Practice

1. 10 minutes of yoga: This practice is slow and grounding. Hold the poses for an extended period. Avoid flow-type practices.

Wind Relieving Pose *(Pavana Muktasana)*

Duration: 10 breaths each side

Benefits: Strengthens the back and abdominal muscles, tones the leg and arm muscles, massages the intestines and other organs in the abdomen, helps with digestion and release of gas, reduces constipation, enhances blood circulation in the hip joints, and releases tension in the lower back

Contraindications: High blood pressure, hyperacidity, hernia, slipped disc, testicle disorder, menstruation, neck and back pain

Instructions:
- Lie on your back with your legs straight, feet together, and arms beside your body.
- Breathe in and, as you exhale, bend your right knee and bring it toward your chest and abdomen.
- Clasp your hands behind your right thigh or shin and gently pull your leg toward your right armpit.
- Hold it there, and take 10 deep, long breaths in and out.
- On your last exhale, release your clasped hands and allow your leg to gently come back to the ground and relax.
- Repeat this pose with the left leg, and then with both legs together.
- You may feel inclined to rock up and down on your spine or roll from side to side a few times and then gently release your arms and legs and relax. Feel the stability of the ground supporting you.

Happy Baby Pose *(Ananda Balasana)*

Duration: 15 breaths

Benefits: Gently stretches inner groin and spine, calms the mind to relieve stress and anxiety

Contraindications: Pregnancy, knee injury, neck injury (support neck with a thick, folded blanket)

Instructions:
- Lie on your back. With an exhale, bend your knees into your belly.
- Inhale, grip the outsides of your feet with your hands (if you have difficulty holding the feet directly with your hands, hold onto a belt looped over the sole of each foot).
- Open your knees slightly wider than your torso, then bring your knees toward your armpits at a 90-degree angle. Position each ankle directly over the knee so that your shins are perpendicular to the floor and your knees.
- Flex through the heels. Gently push your feet up into your hands (or the belts) as you pull your hands down to create resistance.

Legs on a Chair or Legs Up the Wall

Duration: 3 to 4 minutes (set a timer so that you can fully relax and don't have to watch the clock)

Benefits: Relieves tension in the pelvis, belly, low back, and backs of the legs; balances the nervous system; calms the mind; releases subtle mental and physical tension throughout the body

---

Contraindications: This pose is an inversion, so avoid if you have serious eye problems, such as glaucoma. If you have serious neck or back problems, only perform this pose under the supervision of an experienced teacher. If your feet begin to tingle during this pose, bend your knees, touch your soles together, and slide the outer edges of your feet down the wall, bringing your heels close to your pelvis.

I recommend starting with the Legs on a Chair position until you feel very comfortable in the pose, and then try the Legs Up the Wall pose.

Legs on a Chair Instructions:

- Start by placing a blanket or yoga mat in front of the chair you would like to use for support.
- Sit on the blanket and bring your legs onto the chair, and then lower your torso down. The blanket should be under your hips and lower back, up to the bottom of your rib cage.
- You want your knees to be at a 90-degree angle, so make sure the chair you're using is not too low or too high. Then relax your entire body for 3 to 4 minutes.
- When you are ready to come out of the pose, bring your knees toward your chest and roll to one side, relax in the fetal position for a couple of breaths, and then use your hands to press yourself up to a seated position.
- After you have mastered the Legs on a Chair position, try Legs Up the Wall.

Legs Up the Wall Instructions:

- Before beginning this pose, determine your ideal distance from the wall. The distance will vary depending on your height and level of flexibility. If your legs feel stiff or you are tall, move farther away from the wall. If you are flexible and shorter, move closer to the wall.
- Start by sitting sideways with your right side next to the wall. Then in one smooth move, lean back, sweep your legs up to the wall, and bring your upper body and head down to the ground.
- Rotate your body into a comfortable position. Your sit bones do not need to be right against the wall. But your legs should be up the wall, torso perpendicular to the wall, and your neck straight. Bend your knees and press your feet into the wall to adjust your torso into alignment.
- Find a comfortable position where you can relax. Keep your legs relatively firm, just enough to hold them vertically in place. Release the weight of your belly into your torso. Let your eyes soften into the sockets and close your eyes.

- If your feet begin to tingle during this pose, bend your knees, touch your soles together, and slide the outer edges of your feet down the wall, bringing your heels close to your pelvis.
- To come out of the pose, lower your legs to one side. Stay on your side for a few breaths, and come up to sitting with an exhalation.

Corpse Pose *(Savasana)*
Duration: 3 to 4 minutes
Benefits: Calms the mind; relieves stress and mild depression; relaxes the body; alleviates headaches, fatigue, and insomnia; lowers blood pressure
Contraindications: None known
Instructions:
- For this pose, you will need two rolled-up towels.
- To begin, sit on the floor with your knees bent, feet on the floor, and lean back onto your forearms and come all the way down to a lying position.
- Place one rolled-up towel under your knees and the other under your neck.
- Inhale and slowly extend the right leg, then the left, pushing through the heels. Release both legs, softening into the groin. Try to keep the legs angled evenly to the midline of the torso, and let the feet turn out equally.
- Reach your arms toward the ceiling, perpendicular to the floor. Rock slightly from side to side and broaden the back ribs and the shoulder blades away from the spine. Then release the arms to the floor. Rest the backs of the hands on the floor several inches away from your body.
- Soften your face, eyes, and tongue. Let your eyes sink deeply into the sockets.
- Make any final adjustments you need, and then relax and allow yourself to become still.

2. Alternate Nostril Breathing Practice

Duration: 5 to 10 minutes (start with 5 minutes and slowly work your way up)
Benefits: Calms the mind, helps release accumulated tension and fatigue, balances the sympathetic nervous system (fight or flight) with the parasympathetic nervous system (rest and digest)
Contraindications: Colds, flu, fever, menstruation, blocked sinuses
Instructions:
- Gently exhale all the breath.
- Close the right nostril with the thumb of the right hand and inhale slowly

and deeply through the left nostril. When you get to the top of your inhale, close the left nostril with the ring finger or index finger of your right hand.

- Release your thumb, and exhale through the right nostril. Inhale through the right nostril, then close the right nostril with your right thumb and release the finger on your left nostril and exhale through the left nostril.
- You have just completed one round. Continue this practice for 5 minutes.

3. 5 to 10 Minute Yoga Nidra Meditation Practice

Duration: 5 to 10 minutes

Benefits: Relaxes the musculoskeletal system; removes blockages and physical pain; balances the nervous system; increases the production of endorphins; lowers stress hormones; reduces stress, depression, anxiety, insomnia, headaches, fibromyalgia, chronic fatigue, hypertension, and blood sugar

Contraindications: None known

About: Yoga nidra is a comprehensive, profound relaxation technique for relieving emotional stress and tension. It is an old yogic practice that provides deep psychological and physical relaxation while maintaining mental functions. Statistically, the prevalence of anxiety and mood disorders is much higher in those with a vata constitution, so they can significantly benefit from a yoga nidra practice. Research shows that yoga nidra is a useful tool for reducing both the cognitive and physiological symptoms of anxiety. Adults with type 2 diabetes can lower glucose levels with a regular yoga nidra practice. Yoga nidra is also highly recommended for insomnia, so if you have difficulty sleeping, practice yoga nidra before bed.

Yoga nidra is a meditation practice that focuses on scanning the body. To become familiar with yoga nidra, start with an audio recording so that you have verbal cues to keep your attention focused on your body. Once you have listened to the recording a few times, you can mentally work your way through your body on your own. As you place your attention on specific body parts, become aware of that part of the body. Keep yourself alert, but do not concentrate too intensely. Yoga nidra is deeply relaxing, so it's very tempting to fall asleep. Try to remain relaxed yet alert.

Instructions:

- Find a comfortable position, seated, or in corpse pose. Develop an awareness of your body from the top of your head to the tips of your toes. Begin with a few slow, deep belly breaths.
- Become aware of your right side: right thumb, second finger, third finger,

fourth finger, fifth finger, palm of the hand, back of the hand, wrist, lower arm, elbow, upper arm, shoulder, armpit, right waist, right hip, right thigh, kneecap, calf muscle, ankle, heel, sole of the right foot, top of the foot, big toe, second toe, third toe, fourth toe, fifth toe.

- Continue in the same manner with your left side.
- Now become aware of your back. Become aware of your right shoulder blade, left shoulder blade, right buttock, left buttock, spine, and entire back.
- Now shift your attention to your head. Notice the top of the head, forehead, both sides of the head, right eyebrow, left eyebrow, the space between the eyebrows, right eyelid, left eyelid, right eye, left eye, right ear, left ear, right cheek, left cheek, nose, tip of the nose, upper lip, lower lip, chin.
- Shift your attention to the throat, right chest, left chest, middle of the chest, navel, and abdomen.
- Now focus on the entire right leg, move to the left leg, and then both legs together.
- Place your attention on the whole of the right arm, then the left arm, and finally both arms together.
- Move your attention to the whole front of the body, including the abdomen, chest, and legs.
- Pay attention to the whole back of the body, including the shoulders, buttocks, and legs.
- Place your attention on the whole back and front of the body together, and then the whole head.
- Now focus on the whole body. Become aware of your body and visualize it, seeing your body being perfectly still in your room.

It's a good idea to keep a daily log of your relaxation practice. This way, you can check off the days and remember to include it as part of your day. You may also want to note any feelings or sensations that arise during your practice. Remember that it *is* a practice; the first days are the hardest days, and they may feel awkward. But it gets more comfortable, I promise!

DAILY RELAXATION JOURNAL

	Sunday	Monday	Tuesday	Wednesday	Thursday	Friday	Saturday
Week 1							
Week 2							
Week 3							
Week 4							
Week 5							
Week 6							
Week 7							
Week 8							
Week 9							
Week 10							
Week 11							
Week 12							

Exercise

Vata people already have a lot of movement in their constitution, so the vata exercise program includes daily walking for cardiovascular exercise and resistance training for building muscle mass. The vata body type tends to have thin, lean muscles. Vata people can benefit from resistance training to build muscle for glucose uptake. Resistance training includes activities such as using resistance bands, weightlifting, hatha yoga, and Pilates.

WEEKLY EXERCISE PROGRAM

- 120 minutes of resistance training weekly
  - 30 minutes of training four times per week

- 30 minutes of daily walking
  - Three 10-minute walks after meals or 30 minutes daily

If you are new to exercising, start by making slow changes that will last. For some, that may mean walking for 10 minutes after each meal for the first week and then starting the resistance training on the second week. Do what works best for you so that you can continue the exercise program long after the 12-week program.

Resistance Training

One of the best ways for vata people to practice resistance training is with weightlifting. Weightlifting is a critical activity for managing weight loss and balancing blood glucose. Make sure to obtain medical clearance from your healthcare provider before starting a weight-training program. I also recommend starting with a trainer who can provide encouragement and support to prevent injury. Proper clothing and footwear are imperative. Your clothing should be clean and comfortable to avoid chafing. A good quality sneaker with excellent support is essential for stability and balance.

It is crucial to emphasize proper form during weightlifting. Slow, controlled motions are ideal. Avoid fast, wavering movements. Never drop weights; you could hurt yourself or someone else. Avoid locking or overextending your joints. Keep your joints soft to protect your body from strain or injury.

Start slowly, using light weights. Stay with the same weights for the first week or two and increase after that. You may want to start with one set of 10 to 12 repetitions for the first week. The second week, bump up to two sets. Rest for about a minute after the first set, and then repeat the same exercise, with the same number of repetitions. Continue with 1 to 2 sets of appropriate activities for each of the major muscle groups. Working the bigger muscles requires more energy and effort, so it is best to exercise them first while your strength and stamina are high. If there are other specific areas you want to target, focus on those areas after you have worked the major muscle groups.

After a few weeks, you may want to experiment with new exercises. Experimentation will allow you to find the most effective and beneficial routine. You can also add more sets and more weight. As you increase strength, do not sacrifice form. Stick to disciplined alignment in your lifting form.

In the beginning, try to schedule a rest day between workouts. A rest day will allow your muscles to recuperate and get stronger. Eventually, you will get stronger and be able to take on more frequent workouts. The key is to work hard and stay focused, but to always allow ample time for your body to rest. Without proper rest, the body will break down under the continual strain of pushing it.

The following exercises may be particularly helpful for reversing type 2 diabetes:
- Chest press/seated row
- Squats
- Shoulder press/lateral pull
- Leg extension/leg curl
- Abdominal crunch/back extension
- Lateral lift
- Elbow flexion/extension
- Horizontal leg press
- Pectoral deck

After 8 weeks, you will notice significant changes in yourself. You will have more energy and strength, which will bring ease in doing your daily chores and activities. You will start to see a different person looking back at you in the mirror as your body starts to build muscle and burn fat. You may receive compliments from friends and family. All this will bring a feeling of vitality and confidence.

You can go as far as you want with weight training. The benefits of weightlifting are numerous. It improves physical and mental fitness, promotes longevity, manages weight, improves strength and balance, increases bone strength and density, improves sleep, balances blood sugar, and reduces the risk of developing type 2 diabetes and other chronic diseases.

Walking After Meals

Taking a short walk after meals is a highly recommended Ayurvedic practice to promote healthy digestion and prevent type 2 diabetes. The muscle contractions connected with short walks help reduce post-meal glucose levels. Vata people can have quick utilization of glucose by their skeletal muscles, so their walks may be slightly shorter to receive the same benefits as a pitta or kapha person. Vata people should walk for 10 minutes after each meal. Try to stay consistent with your walking schedule, but if you find that you need to skip a walk, increase your next walk to 20 minutes.

It's a good idea to plan your week and log your workouts so that you can keep track of your goals. Please use the chart below, an app, or whatever you need to stay on top of your exercise. The chart below includes a column for each walk and resistance-training session per week. Please check off each column as you complete the exercise. A consistent exercise routine is crucial for the success of the program.

Exercise Journal

	10 min. walk after breakfast	10 min. walk after lunch	10 min. walk after dinner	30 min. resistance	30 min. resistance	30 min. resistance	30 min. resistance
Week 1							
Week 2							
Week 3							
Week 4							
Week 5							
Week 6							
Week 7							
Week 8							
Week 9							
Week 10							
Week 11							
Week 12							

8-Week Supplement Schedule

Please see the Resources section in the back of this book for recommendations on where to purchase your herbs.

1. Barley tea

I recommend that everyone consume this daily. Look for hulled barley (also called Scotch barley) because unlike hull-less or pearl barley, it retains the bran, which delivers fiber in the form of complex carbohydrates.

Makes: about 3 cups

Ingredients:

- 3 cups hot water
- 2 tablespoons hulled barley
- 2 tablespoons almond milk
- ¼ teaspoon ground cinnamon
- ¼ teaspoon ground fenugreek
- ¼ teaspoon ground ginger
- ⅛ teaspoon ground turmeric
- a pinch of black pepper

Instructions: Bring the water to a boil in a saucepan over medium-high heat. Stir in barley, milk, cinnamon, fenugreek, ginger, turmeric, and pepper. Cover and reduce heat to medium-low. Simmer for 3 minutes. Enjoy.

2. Triphala

Recommended if you experience weight gain, gas, bloating, constipation, heaviness after meals, lethargy, thick coating on the tongue, or excess mucus

Dosage: 1 teaspoon at night

3. Bitter melon

Recommended if you experience indigestion, low levels of insulin, or high post-meal blood glucose

Dosage: If you weigh under 200 pounds, ¼ teaspoon after breakfast and dinner. If you weigh over 200 pounds, ½ teaspoon after breakfast and dinner.

4. Tulsi

Recommended if you experience low energy, fatigue, inflammation, pain, swelling, gas and bloating, weight gain, brain fog, or mood swings

Dosage: If you weigh under 200 pounds, ¼ teaspoon before breakfast and dinner.

If you weigh over 200 pounds, ½ teaspoon before breakfast and dinner.

5. Gymnema sylvestre

Recommended if you experience sugar cravings, carbohydrate cravings, overeating, excessive appetite, sluggish digestion, or weight gain

Dosage: If you weigh under 200 pounds, ¼ teaspoon before breakfast and dinner. If you weigh over 200 pounds, ½ teaspoon before breakfast and dinner.

The 12-Week Program: 8-Week Constitution and Elimination Diet for Pitta

The goals for the first 8 weeks of this program include eating meals that calm and balance pitta without being too hot or sweet. Pittas tend to have a lot of body heat and can get "hangry" (hungry + angry), so it's essential to keep mealtimes regular.

The bitter and astringent tastes are particularly beneficial for the pitta person. Bitter is the lightest and coldest of all the tastes. It purifies and dries up secretions, toning the body by reducing excess moisture. The bitter taste is cooling and often associated with reducing inflammation and fever. Bitter is detoxifying and antibacterial, so it is therefore used to cleanse the blood, reduce tumors, and stimulate the liver. Examples of bitter foods include dandelion leaves, bitter greens, aloe vera juice, and bitter melon.

The astringent taste heals, purifies, and constricts all body parts. It tightens and tones the tissues of the body and reduces secretions. Astringent herbs and foods promote healing, alleviate diarrhea, and promote the absorption of fluids. Astringent is anti-inflammatory, antibiotic, antibacterial, and hemostatic (stops bleeding). Examples of astringent foods and herbs include raspberry leaves, pomegranate, dandelion leaves, green beans, cranberries, and leafy green vegetables.

Try to include bitter and astringent tastes in every meal. One of the easiest ways to do this is to add bitter and astringent spices. Cumin, coriander, fennel, turmeric, fenugreek, and ginger make a great combination. You can make a culinary spice blend and use it on all your meals to ensure you are getting bitter and astringent tastes. Also, try to include bitter greens with every meal. Put sautéed bitter greens in an egg-white omelet. For lunch, sauté some spinach and serve it with a grilled chicken breast. Mix a handful of kale into your soup for dinner.

Emphasize a pitta-pacifying diet for the next 8 weeks, including cooling, bitter, and astringent foods. Avoid hot, salty, spicy, or fried foods, especially in the summer. Pitta people can have a robust appetite, so watch your portion sizes and avoid overeating. Eat at regular mealtimes. This will help regulate digestion. Most of your calories should come from vegetables on the pitta food list. Your plate should have about 50 percent vegetables and fruits, 25 percent lean protein, and 25 percent complex carbohydrates and clean fats.

Pitta Food Lists

Fruits to include (sweet or astringent tastes): apples, applesauce, avocados, blackberries, blueberries, cherries, coconuts, elderberries, goji berries, goose berries, grapes, jackfruit (ripe), limes, pomegranates, raspberries, strawberries

Fruits to avoid (sour tastes): grapefruit, lemon, peaches, persimmons, rhubarb

Vegetables to include (cooked): artichokes, arugula, asparagus, beets, bitter melon, black olives, bok choy, broccoli, Brussels sprouts, cabbage, carrots, cauliflower, celery, collard greens, cucumbers, dandelion greens, dulse, fennel, green beans, hijiki, jackfruit (unripe) jicama, kale, kelp, kombu, leafy greens, leeks, lettuce, mushrooms, okra, onions, parsley, parsnips, sweet bell peppers, spaghetti squash, spinach, sprouts, summer squash, taro root, seaweed, winter squash, watercress, zucchini

Vegetables to include in moderation: corn, eggplant

Vegetables to avoid: garlic, horseradish, green olives, onions (raw), peppers (hot), chilis, radishes, tomatoes, turnips, turnip greens

Grains to enjoy: amaranth, barley, black rice, steel-cut oats, quinoa, wild rice

Grains to avoid: brown rice, buckwheat, millet, wheat, polenta, rye

Legumes to enjoy: azuki beans, black beans, black-eyed peas, chickpeas (garbanzo beans), kidney beans, black lentils, brown lentils, lima beans, mung beans, mung dal, navy beans, green peas, pinto beans, red lentils, soybeans, split peas, tempeh, tofu

Legumes to avoid: black lentils, pigeon peas

Dairy to enjoy: ghee

Dairy to avoid: hard cheese, feta cheese, ice cream, all animal milk, sour cream, yogurt

Meat and eggs to enjoy: chicken (white meat), turkey (white meat), venison, egg whites

Meat and eggs to avoid: beef, chicken (dark meat), turkey (dark meat), duck, lamb, pork, seafood, egg yolk

Nuts to enjoy: almonds

Nuts to avoid: brazil nuts, cashews, filberts/hazelnuts, macadamia nuts, peanuts, pecans, pine nuts, pistachios, walnuts

Seeds to enjoy: flax, hemp, pumpkin, sunflower

Seeds to avoid: chia, sesame

Oils to enjoy (organic, cold-pressed): avocado, almond, coconut, flaxseed, ghee, olive, primrose, sunflower, walnut

Oils to avoid: apricot, corn, sesame, safflower

Spices to enjoy: basil (fresh), cardamom, cinnamon, coriander, cumin, fennel, fenugreek, ginger (fresh), parsley, saffron, tarragon, turmeric, vanilla, wintergreen

Spices to avoid (hot): allspice, anise, black pepper, caraway, cayenne, chili pepper, cloves, garlic, horseradish, mustard seeds, nutmeg, paprika, poppy seeds

Beverages to enjoy: almond milk, aloe vera juice, unsweetened soft cider, barley tea, coconut milk, coconut water, rose water, unsweetened pomegranate juice

Beverages to enjoy in moderation: black tea, chai

Beverages to avoid: alcohol, sour berry juice, carbonated drinks, coffee, carrot juice, cranberry juice, grapefruit juice, iced drinks, lemonade, orange juice, pungent teas, salted drinks

Herbs to enjoy: aloe vera, blackberry, burdock, catnip, chamomile, chicory, cilantro, dandelion, dill, hibiscus, hops, jasmine, kukicha, lavender, lemon balm, lemongrass, licorice, marshmallow, mint, nettle, oat straw, passionflower, raspberry leaf, red clover, sarsaparilla, strawberry leaf, yarrow

Herbs to avoid: bay leaf, marjoram, oregano, parsley, rosemary, sage, sassafras, savory, tarragon, thyme, yerba mate

Condiments to enjoy: coconut, liquid amino acids

Condiments to avoid (sour): mustard, tahini, mayonnaise, pickles, sauerkraut, soy sauce, vinegar

Recipes for Pitta

BASIC PITTA RECIPES

GOLDEN COCONUT MILK

Coconut milk is a cool, refreshing brain tonic. This beverage will help soothe your nervous system as you unwind from the day. Add a pinch of fresh nutmeg and drink before bed to promote restful sleep.

Makes: Four 8-ounce servings

Ingredients:

- 2 cups water
- 1 can (14 ounces) coconut milk
- ¼ teaspoon ghee (see page 164)
- ¼ teaspoon ground turmeric
- Pinch of ground cinnamon

Instructions:

1. Combine water and coconut milk in a saucepan. Add ghee and bring to a simmer over medium-high heat.
2. Whisk in turmeric and cinnamon and simmer, stirring occasionally, for 3 minutes. Set aside to cool. Pour into four cups or mugs.

MUNG BEAN DIP

Lightly spiced and adaptable to use as a dip with raw vegetables or as a spread, this dish is a healthy addition to pitta-friendly snacks and main dishes.

Makes: about 2 cups

Ingredients:

- 1 cup dried mung beans, well rinsed
- Pinch of hing/asafetida (see headnote, page 79)
- ¼ teaspoon ground cumin
- ¼ teaspoon dried dill
- 2 tablespoons freshly squeezed lime juice
- ½ cup extra-virgin olive oil

Instructions:

1. The night before, cover beans with 3 cups of water in a large pot. Add hing

and set aside to soak overnight.

2. The next day, drain and rinse beans in a colander. Combine beans, ¼ cup water, cumin, and dill in a food processor. Process for 20 seconds. With the motor running, add lime juice through the funnel in the lid. Keep the motor running and add the oil slowly.

CILANTRO PESTO

Cilantro is a wonderful cooling and detoxifying addition to meals. It reduces inflammation in the urinary tract and removes heavy metals from the bloodstream.

Makes: 2 ½ cups

Ingredients:

- ¼ cup raw almonds
- 1 ripe avocado, flesh cut into quarters
- 2 cups coarsely chopped fresh cilantro
- ½ cup coarsely chopped fresh parsley
- 3 tablespoons freshly squeezed lime juice
- 4 to 6 tablespoons extra-virgin olive oil

Instructions:

1. Add almonds to a food processor. Process for 30 seconds or until coarsely chopped. Add avocado and process for 20 seconds.

2. Add cilantro and parsley to the food processor and sprinkle lime juice on top. With the motor running, slowly add 4 tablespoons of the oil through the funnel in the lid and process for about 1 minute, stopping to scrape down the sides and to check on the consistency of the pesto. For a smoother, thinner consistency, add the remaining oil.

PITTA BREAKFAST

COCONUT-BERRY OVERNIGHT OATMEAL BOWL

Serve this easy breakfast bowl with a cup of blackberries, blueberries, cherries, or gooseberries.

Makes: 1 serving

Ingredients:

- ½ cup coconut milk
- ½ cup steel-cut oats
- 1 tablespoon shredded, unsweetened coconut
- 1 tablespoon chopped raw almonds
- 1 cup of berries (see headnote, above)

Instructions:

1. Combine milk and oats in a bowl. Cover and set in the refrigerator overnight.
2. In the morning, remove from refrigerator and transfer into a small, lightly oiled saucepan. Stir in shredded coconut and warm over medium heat, stirring constantly, for 1 minute or until warmed through. Serve hot or warm with almonds and berries sprinkled on top.

Alternative method—use a double boiler: To save a step and make this oil-free, combine milk, oats, and coconut in the top of a double boiler. Cover and refrigerate. In the morning, bring an inch of water in the bottom of the double boiler to a boil. Fit the top boiler over the bottom, cover, and heat, stirring frequently, for 1 minute or until warmed through. If you do not have a double boiler, a heatproof bowl that fits over a saucepan (but does not touch the bottom of the pan) will work just as well.

BREAKFAST BOWL WITH GOLDEN MILK

For a savory snack, breakfast, or lunch bowl, substitute chopped artichoke, asparagus, cucumber, shredded carrot, or daikon radish for the berries and apple.

Makes: 4 to 6 servings

Ingredients:

- 2 cups water
- 1 cup black rice
- ½ cup goji berries or quartered fresh strawberries
- 1 apple, chopped
- 1 can (14 ounces) coconut milk
- 1 teaspoon ground turmeric
- ½ teaspoon ground cardamom
- ½ teaspoon ground cinnamon
- ¼ cup shredded, unsweetened coconut

Instructions:

1. Bring water to a boil in a saucepan over high heat. Stir in rice, cover, and reduce heat to medium-low. Simmer for 55 minutes. Turn heat off and quickly stir in berries and apple. Cover and let sit on the burner for 5 minutes. Remove lid, stir, and set aside.
2. Combine milk, turmeric, cardamom, and cinnamon in a saucepan. Bring to a simmer over medium heat, whisking constantly for 3 minutes or until small bubbles appear around the edges of the pan. Remove from heat.
3. Spoon rice and fruit into serving bowls and pour milk on top. Sprinkle coconut on top and serve warm.

BROCCOLI MUSHROOM SCRAMBLE

Egg yolk can be too heating for pitta, so make your scrambles with egg whites only. Broccoli is packed with nutrients and is high in fiber. And when combined with egg whites and mushrooms, it creates a high-protein breakfast that will keep you satiated until lunch.

Makes: 2 servings

Ingredients:

- 1 tablespoon extra-virgin avocado oil or ghee (see page 164)
- 1 cup chopped broccoli
- ½ cup chopped mushrooms
- 4 egg whites

Instructions:

Heat oil in a skillet over medium-low heat. Add broccoli and mushrooms and cook, stirring frequently, for 4 minutes. Add egg whites and cook, stirring constantly, for about 5 minutes or until cooked through.

PANCAKES AND FRUIT

The chickpea flour adds plant protein and is a good choice for pancakes because it emulsifies and keeps the pancakes from breaking during cooking.

Makes: 4 pancakes

Ingredients:

- 1 cup chickpea flour
- ¼ cup finely chopped raw almonds
- 1 teaspoon baking soda
- ¾ cup almond milk or coconut milk
- 2 tablespoons applesauce
- 1 tablespoon ghee (see page 164), or more as needed
- 1 cup any of the following: fresh blueberries, cherries, goji berries, strawberries

Instructions:

1. In a large bowl, combine flour, almonds, and baking soda. In a 2-cup measuring cup, measure milk and stir in applesauce. Slowly add the milk mixture to the chickpea mixture, mixing just until all of the dry ingredients are incorporated into the batter (there may be small lumps).

2. Heat ghee in a large, heavy (cast iron if possible) skillet over medium-high heat. Using a ½-cup measure, scoop out the batter and scrape into a mound in the skillet. Measure 2 or 3 more mounds of batter into the skillet. Cook for 2 minutes or until the edges start to show a golden color. Flip the pancakes and cook for another 2 minutes or until lightly browned on the opposite side.

3. Add another tablespoon of ghee if needed, and repeat step 1 with any

remaining batter. Serve the pancakes warm, topped with fresh fruit.

ZUCCHINI KALE SCRAMBLE

Zucchini is a versatile, mild-tasting vegetable. It can be spiraled into a noodle, grilled, or lightly sautéed. Zucchini is a low-calorie and easy-to-digest food, good for breakfast, lunch, or dinner.

Makes: 2 servings

Ingredients:

- 1 tablespoon extra-virgin olive oil or ghee (see page 164)
- 1 cup chopped kale
- ½ zucchini, chopped
- ¼ onion, finely chopped
- 4 egg whites

Instructions:

Heat oil in a skillet over medium-low heat. Add kale, zucchini, and onion and cook, stirring frequently, for 3 or 4 minutes or until onion is transparent. Add egg whites and cook, stirring occasionally, for about 5 minutes or until cooked through.

PITTA LUNCH

VEGETABLE COINS WITH CHICKEN AND AVOCADO DRIZZLE

To achieve the thinly sliced vegetables needed for this recipe, I recommend using a mandoline slicer if possible. As a variation, you could use any of the following: 1 cup shaved Brussels sprouts, 1 cup chopped cabbage, 1 cup chopped bell pepper, or 1 cup sliced green beans in place of the carrots, zucchini, and eggplant.

Makes: 4 servings

Ingredients:

Coins

- 1 large carrot
- 1 medium zucchini
- 1 small Japanese eggplant
- 2 cups cooked chicken pieces
- 2 tablespoons ghee (see page 164) or extra-virgin olive oil

Avocado Drizzle

- Juice of ½ lime
- 2 avocados, diced
- 3 tablespoons roasted garlic, optional (see page 76)
- about 4 tablespoons extra-virgin avocado (or other pitta-friendly) oil

Instructions:

1. Peel carrots, zucchini, and eggplant and then slice them crosswise into thin coins using a chef's knife or mandoline slicer.
2. Heat ghee in a large skillet over medium-high heat. Add coins and cook, tossing frequently, for 7 minutes or until crisp-tender. Add chicken and cook, stirring constantly, for 2 minutes or until heated through.
3. Make the drizzle by combining lime juice, avocados, and garlic (if using) in a small bowl. Mash with a fork. Add oil 1 tablespoon at a time until a thin consistency is achieved.
4. Divide vegetable/chicken mixture into four equal portions and pile on plates. Drizzle each with avocado mixture.

CHICKEN DELUXE SALAD

Raw foods are a little harder to digest than cooked foods. Try to consume salads and other raw foods for lunch, when your digestive fire is at its strongest.

Makes: 2 to 3 servings

Ingredients:

- 1 tablespoon extra-virgin avocado oil or ghee (see page 164)
- 1 boneless, skinless chicken breast, coarsely chopped
- 1 head Boston lettuce
- ½ cup shredded carrot
- ½ cup chopped cucumber
- ½ cup chopped celery
- 1 hardboiled egg white, sliced or chopped
- ½ cup avocado drizzle (see page 108)

Instructions:

1. Heat oil in a small skillet over medium heat. Add chicken and cook, stirring frequently, for 1 minute or until browned on each side. Add enough water to the pan to cover the chicken pieces. Cover the pan, lower the heat to medium-low, and simmer for 5 to 7 minutes or until the center of the chicken turns opaque and the internal temperature reaches 165° F. Drain and set chicken aside to cool slightly.
2. Shred or chop lettuce and transfer to a salad bowl. Add carrot, cucumber, celery, egg white, and chicken pieces and toss to mix well. Pour avocado drizzle on top and toss to mix.

ZUCCHINI TURKEY BURGERS

Turkey burgers are a great replacement for beef burgers. For variety, swap out the zucchini for fennel bulb, celery, or artichoke.

Makes: 4 burgers
Ingredients:

- 1pound ground white turkey breast
- 1 large zucchini, shredded
- ½ teaspoon chopped fresh dill
- ½ teaspoon ground fenugreek
- about 2 tablespoons extra-virgin coconut oil
- lettuce cups

Instructions:

1. Combine turkey, zucchini, dill, and fenugreek in a food processor. Process on high for 2 minutes or until the mixture is smooth and holds together.
2. Lightly oil the palms of your hands and form the mixture into four patties.
3. Heat 1 tablespoon of oil in a large skillet over medium heat. Cook the patties for about 3 to 4 minutes on each side, or until golden brown and cooked through. Turkey is cooked when the internal temperature reaches 165° F. Serve between two lettuce cups.

TURKEY WITH PARSNIPS AND GREEN BEANS

Kelp is a great addition to any slow-cooker meal. It is a superfood and is great for all constitutions. It helps reduce blood sugar spikes and, when used in a bone broth, it extracts more minerals from the bones.

Makes: 6 servings
Ingredients:

- 1 cup (or more) vegetable broth or water
- 1 teaspoon ground fenugreek
- ½ teaspoon kelp
- ½ teaspoon ground turmeric
- 3 cups very coarsely chopped green beans
- 3 cups sliced parsnips
- ½ small turkey, bone-in

Instructions:

1. Mix broth, fenugreek, kelp, and turmeric in a large slow cooker. Add beans and parsnips.
2. Cut turkey into 3 or 4 pieces and remove skin. Place turkey in the slow cooker, nestling the pieces into the vegetables. Add more broth if needed to cover the turkey. Set temperature to low or medium, cover, and cook for 6 to 8 hours or until the internal temperature of a large turkey piece reaches 165° F.
3. Lift out turkey and cool slightly. Remove bones, cut meat into small pieces, and return to the liquid before serving.

PITTA VEGETABLE-MUNG BEAN POTS WITH SEED CRUST

The seed crust is crunchy and makes a tasty topping for this bean-and-vegetable stew. Fresh fennel bulb adds a hint of anise (licorice) flavor to the dish, but it's if not available, you can use 1 cup of chopped cabbage or cauliflower in its place. Be sure to use ovenproof pots or ramekins for this oven-baked dish.

Makes: 4 servings

Ingredients:

Bean Pots

- 1 ½ cups water or vegetable stock
- ½ cup split dried mung beans, well rinsed
- 2 tablespoons ghee (see page 164), divided
- ½ fennel bulb, chopped (about 1 cup, see note above)
- 1 carrot, finely chopped
- 1 celery stalk, chopped
- 1 small zucchini, chopped
- 1 cup coconut milk

Seed Crust

- ½ cup cooked wild rice
- ¼ cup raw sunflower seeds
- 2 tablespoons raw pumpkin seeds
- 1 tablespoon flaxseeds
- about 3 tablespoons extra-virgin almond oil

Instructions:

1. Bring water to a boil in a saucepan over high heat. Add beans, cover, reduce heat to medium-low, and simmer for 25 minutes or just until tender. Drain and combine with 1 tablespoon ghee in a bowl. Set aside.

2. Preheat oven to 375° F. Place four heatproof ramekins or small, ovenproof bowls on a baking sheet and set aside.

3. Meanwhile, heat remaining ghee in a large skillet over medium-high heat. Add fennel, carrot, celery, and zucchini and cook, stirring frequently, for 7 minutes or until vegetables are crisp-tender. Stir in milk and simmer, stirring constantly, for 1 minute. Remove from heat and stir in cooked beans. Spoon the mixture into the four ramekins.

4. To make the seed crust, combine rice and seeds in a food processor. With the motor running, add oil through the funnel in the lid until the mixture starts to clump together. Divide crust mixture into 4 equal portions and pat over vegetable mixture in ramekins. Bake in preheated oven for 20 minutes or until the bean mixture is bubbling and the crust is lightly browned.

CREAMY RED LENTIL VEGGIE SOUP

Red lentils create a thick, creamy soup base and are fantastic for reducing blood sugar. Replace potatoes with red lentils to create rich, delicious soups and side dishes.

Makes: 4 servings

Ingredients:

- 1 tablespoon ghee (see page 164) or extra-virgin sunflower oil
- 1 ½ teaspoons ground coriander
- ½ teaspoon ground fennel
- ½ cup red lentils
- 1 teaspoon grated fresh ginger
- 1 cup chopped cabbage
- 1 cup chopped asparagus
- 1 cup chopped broccoli
- 4 cups water

Instructions:

Heat ghee in a skillet over medium-high heat. Add coriander and fennel and cook, stirring frequently, for 3 to 5 minutes or until brown. Add red lentils and ginger and cook, stirring frequently, for 2 to 3 minutes. Stir in cabbage, asparagus, and broccoli. Add water and bring to a boil. Reduce heat to medium and cook, stirring occasionally, for 30 minutes or until vegetables are tender.

SPIRALED ZUCCHINI WITH JACKFRUIT AND CILANTRO PESTO

Unripe jackfruit is frequently used in Ayurvedic dishes to help balance type 2 diabetes. It has a neutral taste that absorbs the flavors around it. Try using it as a replacement for chicken, tofu, or turkey.

Makes: 4 servings

Ingredients:

- 4 zucchini, cut into spirals
- 1 cup chopped unripe jackfruit, fresh, frozen, or canned
- ½ cup chopped mushrooms
- 1 tablespoon extra-virgin avocado oil or ghee (see page 164)
- ¼ cup cilantro pesto (see page 105)

Instructions:

Heat oil in a large skillet over medium heat. Add zucchini, jackfruit, and mushrooms and cook, stirring frequently, for 10 minutes or until zucchini and jackfruit are crisp-tender. Stir in pesto and heat through.

CREAMY BROCCOLI SOUP

This quick, easy-to-digest soup makes a perfect lunch or dinner. Swap out the broccoli for celery, cauliflower, asparagus, or carrots to make a variety of creamy soups.

Makes: 2 servings

Ingredients:

- 2 cups bone broth
- 4 cups chopped broccoli florets and tender stems (1 or 2 large heads broccoli)
- 1 avocado, coarsely chopped
- 1 tablespoon chopped fresh dill or 1 teaspoon dried

Instructions:

1. Bring broth to a boil in a saucepan over high heat, and then reduce to a simmer. Add the broccoli and simmer, stirring occasionally, for 7 to 8 minutes or until crisp-tender.
2. Reduce heat to low. Add avocado and dill to the saucepan and warm through.
3. Transfer soup to a blender. Cover and purée on high, about 1 minute or until smooth.

BLACK BEAN BOWL

The American Diabetes Association recommends regularly including beans in the diet to reduce blood glucose. Pitta people have the digestive strength to handle most types of beans. For variety, swap out the black beans for any other bean on the pitta food list. If purchasing canned beans, look for BPA-free tins and no sodium added.

Makes: 4 to 6 servings

Ingredients:

- 1 tablespoon ghee (see page 164) or extra-virgin avocado oil
- ¼ teaspoon ground coriander
- ⅛ teaspoon ground turmeric
- 1 can (15 ounces) black beans, drained and rinsed
- 1 cup chopped firm tofu
- 1 cup chopped kale
- 1 avocado, chopped
- 1 jicama, chopped
- ½ cup chopped fresh cilantro
- Juice of 1 lime

Instructions:

1. In a large saucepan, heat ghee over medium heat. Add coriander and turmeric and cook, stirring constantly, for 30 seconds. Add beans, tofu, and

kale. Cook, stirring constantly, for about 5 minutes or until kale is tender. Remove from heat and transfer to a bowl.

2. Add avocado, jicama, cilantro, and lime juice and toss well to combine. Serve warm.

CAULIFLOWER LIME RICE

Cauliflower rice makes a great substitute for grains. Eat it alone for a light dinner or serve it with chicken, turkey, or jackfruit for a hearty lunch.

Makes: 4 to 6 servings

Ingredients:

- 1 small head cauliflower
- 1 tablespoon ghee (see page 164) or extra-virgin coconut oil
- ¼ teaspoon ground coriander
- ¼ teaspoon ground turmeric
- ½ cup fresh or canned (drained) artichoke hearts
- 3 tablespoons chopped fresh dill
- 2 tablespoons lime zest

Instructions:

1. Trim cauliflower and place florets in a blender (you may have to do this in batches). Pulse until chopped to the size of rice grains. Transfer to a bowl and set aside.

2. Heat ghee in a large skillet over medium-high heat. Add coriander, turmeric, and artichokes and cook, stirring frequently, for about 5 minutes or until the artichokes are browned.

3. Stir in cauliflower rice, reduce heat to medium and cook, stirring frequently, for 6 to 8 minutes or until cauliflower is crisp-tender. Stir in dill and lime zest, and heat through.

Sleep Optimization

Pitta people do best with a moderate amount of sleep—about 7 to 8 hours. They may have difficulty falling asleep, but once asleep they can usually stay asleep. Sleeplessness for pitta people is usually due to stress, hostility, or overheating. Pitta people have more acidity and inflammatory issues associated with their imbalances. They may develop gastric ulcers, sour belching, and inflammation in the digestive system, so for a good night's sleep it's important for them to stay away from heavy, fried foods (especially for dinner, as they will cause distress throughout the night).

Pitta people must meditate daily and talk about their issues as they arise. When they are out of balance, they can become angry, and anger will only make their inflammation worse. If they go to bed angry, they are going to have a sleepless night. Pitta people need to practice empathy, compassion, and forgiveness to stay balanced. Before going to bed, make sure the room is cool and comfortable. Make a list of all the things you are thinking about and what you want to accomplish tomorrow. Remove all electronics, screens, and lights from the bedroom. While in bed, think about things from the day for which you are grateful, and let your body rest. If you are unable to sleep, practice progressive muscle relaxation.

Progressive muscle relaxation was developed in the 1930s by the American physician Edmund Jacobson. Based on the premise that mental calmness is a natural result of physical relaxation, progressive muscle relaxation is a deep relaxation technique used to control insomnia-related stress and anger. Progressive muscle relaxation is the simple practice of tensing, or tightening, a group of muscles and then releasing and relaxing them. This process works very well for removing anger and stress from the body. When we experience these emotions, we often also have physical tension, unbeknownst to us. By constricting and releasing specific muscles, you can discover where you are holding tension and consciously release it. Relaxing the body will calm the mind, facilitating sleep.

Progressive Muscle Relaxation

- Lie on your back and close your eyes.
- Feel your feet. Sense their weight. On an inhale, contract the muscles of your feet and, on an exhale, relax your feet and allow them to sink into the bed. Start with your toes and progress to your ankles and calves.
- Feel your knees. Sense their weight. On an inhale, contract the muscles around your knees and, on an exhale, relax your knees and feel them sink into the bed.
- Feel your upper legs and thighs. Feel their weight. On an inhale, contract the muscles of your upper legs and, on an exhale, relax your upper legs and feel them sink into the bed.
- Feel your abdomen and chest. Sense your breathing. Consciously let your muscles relax. Deepen your breath slightly and feel your belly. On an inhale, contract the abdominal muscles and, on an exhale, release your abdominal muscles and sink into the bed.
- Feel your buttocks. Sense their weight. On an inhale, contract the muscles of your buttocks and, on an exhale, relax your buttocks and feel them sink into the bed.
- Feel your hands. Sense their weight. On an inhale, contract the muscles in your hands and, on an exhale, relax your hands and feel them sink into the bed.

- Feel your forearms. Sense their weight. On an inhale, contract the muscles and, on an exhale, relax them and feel them sink into the bed.
- Feel your upper arms. Sense their weight. On an inhale, contract the muscles in your upper arms and, on an exhale, relax them and feel them sink into the bed.
- Feel your shoulders. Sense their weight. On an inhale, contract the shoulder muscles and, on an exhale, relax them and feel them sink into the bed.
- Feel your neck. Sense its weight. On an inhale, contract the muscles in your neck and, on an exhale, relax and feel your neck sink into the bed.
- Feel your head. Sense its weight. On an inhale, contract the muscles in your head and, on an exhale, consciously relax them and feel your head sink into the bed.
- Feel your mouth and jaw. Consciously relax that area. Pay particular attention to your jaw muscles and unclench them if you need to. Feel your mouth and jaw relax and sink into the bed.
- Feel your eyes. Sense if there is tension in your eyes. On an inhale, close your eyes. On an exhale, consciously relax your eyelids and feel the tension slide off the eyes.
- Feel your face and cheeks. On an inhale, contract your facial muscles and, on an exhale, relax them and feel the tension slide off into the bed.
- Mentally scan your body. If you find any place that is still tense, contract those muscles on an inhale and, on an exhale, relax that area and let it sink into the bed.

Lifestyle Enhancement

Pitta people like organization and structure, and they thrive when they are on a schedule. They can benefit from moderate exercise. You may want to push yourself too hard, so be mindful to exercise within your capacity to avoid injury. If you haven't exercised in a while, start out slowly and increase your activity level over the 8 weeks.

Pitta Daily Schedule

Wake up: 4:00–5:00 a.m.
30 minutes of exercise
Breakfast: 7:00–8:00 a.m.
10-minute walk
Lunch: 12:00–1:00 p.m.
10-minute walk

Dinner: 6:00–7:00 p.m.
10-minute walk
30-minute relaxation practice
Go to sleep: 9:00–10:00 p.m.

When pitta people get out of balance, they tend to have difficulty dealing with anger and heat, so the lifestyle-enhancement program for pittas emphasizes the importance of anger management and heat reduction. When a pitta person becomes irritated, they may feel confrontational and begin picking fights. They can become judgmental and lack patience and tolerance. They can become easily irritated or aggressive and show domineering behavior. If this happens to you, try to relax and avoid the factors that cause aggravation. Anything that heats the body up will irritate pitta. Summertime can be especially challenging for pitta people. The hot summer sun can set a person's pitta ablaze. Avoid being out in the sun during peak hours of the day. Try to stay in cool, shaded areas. Competitive sports can also really provoke anger in a pitta person. Try to engage in exercise with people who are not competitive.

30-Minute Daily Relaxation Practice

The best way to calm pitta is with a daily relaxation practice. Allow 30 minutes for your practice. It includes yoga poses, breathwork, and meditation. If you are new to these practices, don't be afraid to give them a try. The yoga poses are gentle and restorative. Yoga has been shown to improve sleep length and quality. The recommended breathwork is soothing, and you may notice an immediate effect. The meditation is a simple exercise that you can do on your own or with guided audio.

Try to include your relaxation practice as a daily routine. Aim for 30 minutes, but if you can't get 30 minutes in and can only do 10 minutes, please do it for 10 minutes. A little is better than nothing, and consistency is more beneficial than irregularity. Once you begin to explore your relaxation practice, you may find that you gravitate toward one activity over another. If that happens, feel free to alter the times spent in each activity. You may also want to use a timer so that you can fully relax in each practice and not watch the clock.

1. 15 minutes of yoga poses: This practice is slow and grounding, involving a gentle flow and holding poses for an extended period. It includes seated twists, forward bends, and restorative poses.

Cat/Cow Pose

Duration: 3 to 4 minutes

Benefits: Massages the organs, improves kidney function, balances emotions, relieves stress, calms the mind

Contraindications: Neck injury

Instructions: Start on your hands and knees in a "tabletop" position. Make sure that your knees are directly below your hips and that your wrists, elbows, and shoulders are in line and perpendicular to the floor. Center your head in a neutral position, eyes looking at the floor. As you exhale, round your spine toward the ceiling, making sure to keep your shoulders and knees in position. Release your head toward the floor, but don't force your chin to your chest. This is cat pose. On an inhale, relax your belly toward the mat and arch your back. Lift your chin and chest, and gaze up toward the ceiling. Broaden across your shoulder blades and draw your shoulders away from your ears. This is cow pose. Flow from cat to cow pose with each inhale and exhale, coordinating the movement with your own breath. Continue, moving your whole spine. After your final exhale, come back to the neutral tabletop position where you started and notice the effects.

Extended-Leg Forward Bend *(Paschimatanasana)*

Duration: 3 to 4 minutes

Benefits: Calms the mind, reduces stress and anxiety, stimulates the liver, improves digestion

Contraindications: Slipped disc

Instructions: Sit on the floor with your legs straight in front of you. Press actively through your heels and flex your feet. Gently press your thighs into the floor. Place your hands on the floor beside your hips. Keep your chest lifted. Exhale and lean forward from your hip joints, not your waist. Lengthen your tailbone away from the back of your pelvis. Let your arms reach toward your feet and let them rest on your legs without straining yourself. With each inhalation, lift and lengthen your torso slightly; with each exhalation, release a little deeper into the forward bend. Stay in the pose anywhere from 1 to 3 minutes. To release the pose, exhale and lift your torso away from your thighs.

Reclined, Supported Bound Angle Pose *(Baddha Konasana)*

Duration: 3 to 4 minutes

Benefits: Improves digestion, calms the mind, relaxes the nervous system

Contraindications: Groin or knee injury

Instructions: Use blankets and pillows to support your body so you can fully relax in the pose. You will need two pillows, one to go under each knee, and another blanket or pillow to go under your back. As you get into the pose, have the pillows and blankets within reach. Start by sitting on the floor, with your legs and spine straight. Place a pillow or blanket on the floor behind your buttocks. Place your hands in the inner creases of your knees and bend your legs toward your groin. Let your knees fall outward toward the floor. Gently let your thighs fall open and keep your feet together. Carefully place a pillow under each knee. When you have your knees in a comfortable position, slowly lean back on the pillow behind you. Rest your arms alongside your body with palms facing up. Enjoy some deep breathing and relax.

Wind Relieving Pose (Pavana Muktasana)
Duration: 10 breaths each side
Benefits: Strengthens the back and abdominal muscles, tones the leg and arm muscles, massages the intestines and other organs in the abdomen, helps with digestion and release of gas, enhances blood circulation in the hip joints, and releases tension in the lower back
Contraindications: High blood pressure, heart problems, hyperacidity, hernia, slipped disc, testicle disorder, menstruation, neck and back problems
Instructions:
- Lie on your back with your legs straight, feet together, and arms beside your body.
- Breathe in and, as you exhale, bend your right knee and bring it toward your chest and abdomen.
- Clasp your hands behind your right thigh or shin and gently pull your leg toward your right armpit.
- Hold it there, and take 10 deep, long breaths in and out.
- On your last exhale, release your clasped hands and allow your leg to gently come back to the ground and relax.

Repeat this pose with the left leg, and then with both legs together.

You may feel inclined to rock up and down on your spine or roll from side to side a few times and then gently release your arms and legs and relax. Feel the stability of the ground supporting you.

Corpse Pose (Savasana)
Duration: 3 to 4 minutes
Benefits: Calms the mind; relieves stress and mild depression; relaxes the body; alleviates headaches, fatigue, and insomnia; lowers blood pressure

Contraindications: None known

Instructions:

- For this pose, you will need two rolled-up towels, pillows, or blankets.
- To begin, sit on the floor with your knees bent, feet on the floor, and lean back onto your forearms and come all the way down to a lying position.
- Place one rolled-up towel under your knees and the other under your neck.
- Inhale and slowly extend the right leg, then the left, pushing through the heels. Release both legs, softening into the groin. Try to keep the legs angled evenly to the midline of the torso, and let the feet turn out equally.
- Reach your arms toward the ceiling, perpendicular to the floor. Rock slightly from side to side and broaden the back ribs and the shoulder blades away from the spine. Then release the arms to the floor. Rest the backs of the hands on the floor several inches away from your body.
- Soften your face, eyes, and tongue. Let your eyes sink deeply into the sockets.
- Make any final adjustments you need, and then relax and allow yourself to become still.

2. 10-Minute Breathwork: "Humming bee breath," also known as *bhramari*, is a calming breathing practice that soothes the nervous system and releases energy stuck in the throat. This is great for people who have difficulty expressing their emotions. This breathwork produces a humming sound at the back of the throat—just like a buzzing bee. The vibrations created also help stimulate the thyroid, which can help with hypothyroid conditions that cause weight gain and fatigue.

Benefits: Reduces stress, anger, and frustration; lowers blood pressure; stimulates the thyroid; supports pituitary and pineal glands; promotes restful sleep

Contraindications: Ear infection, pregnancy, menstruation, epilepsy, extremely high blood pressure

Instructions:

- Sit in a comfortable, meditative pose. Keep your spine erect. Do not do this lying down.
- Breathe normally and relax your whole body.
- Keep your mouth closed and teeth apart.
- Plug both your ears with your thumbs, gently rest your pointer fingers over your eyes, relax your middle fingers over each nostril, place your ring fingers over your top lip and your pinky fingers over your bottom lip, and close your eyes.
- Take a slow, deep breath and fill your lungs fully.

- Then exhale slowly, gently constricting the back of your throat to make a continuous humming sound. The tone should reverberate in your head. Feel the vibration and be aware of the continuous drone, similar to the buzzing of a bee.
- You have now completed one round. Slowly inhale and repeat.

3. Tratak Meditation with a Candle Flame
Duration: 7 minutes
Benefits: Strengthens the eyes, relieves anxiety and depression, promotes restful sleep, improves concentration
Contraindications: Glaucoma, migraine, epilepsy
Instructions:
- Place a candle about an arm's length away, with the wick of the candle at chest height.
- Light the candle and sit in a comfortable position with a straight spine.
- Practice tratak with your glasses removed. You may have to adjust the distance between the candle and yourself so that you can observe a clear image of the candle wick without blur.
- The flame has three zones of color. At the base of the wick is a reddish color; this is the brightest, most stable part. Keep your eyes fixed on this part of the flame, without blinking.
- Keep your gaze constant.
- When your eyes need a rest, close them. With your eyes closed, observe the image of the flame in your mind's eye. If you don't see it, don't be disappointed—you will start visualizing it with practice. Keep your eyes closed for as long as you see the mental image. Then repeat.

It's a good idea to keep a daily log of your relaxation practice. This way, you can check off the days and remember to include it in your schedule. You may also want to note any feelings or sensations that arise during your practice. Remember that it *is* a practice; the first days are the hardest days, and they may feel awkward. But it gets more comfortable, I promise!

DAILY RELAXATION JOURNAL

	Sunday	Monday	Tuesday	Wednesday	Thursday	Friday	Saturday
Week 1							
Week 2							
Week 3							
Week 4							
Week 5							
Week 6							
Week 7							
Week 8							
Week 9							
Week 10							
Week 11							
Week 12							

Weekly Exercise

The pitta exercise program includes regular walking, resistance training, and cardio workouts. Pitta people already have fire in their constitution, so their exercise program should not be too heating or cause overexertion. Exercise during the coolest part of the day and out of direct sunlight.

Base your activities on enjoyment rather than competition. There are many different forms of exercise you can try—choose ones that you find fulfilling and fun. You will be much happier while you are exercising and more likely to continue. If you decide to try an activity that is new to you, I recommend starting with a trainer. A trainer can help modify alignment, prevent injury, and get you motivated.

By the end of the eighth week of the program, your weekly exercise program should look like this:

WEEKLY EXERCISE PROGRAM

- 120 minutes of weekly exercise
  - 30 minutes of resistance training twice a week
  - 30 minutes of cardiovascular exercise twice a week

- 30 minutes of daily walking
  - Three 10-minute walks after meals or 30 minutes daily

Resistance Training

- **Weightlifting** should include exercises for all muscle groups. Do two to three sets of eight to fifteen repetitions per exercise. Include two leg-extensor exercises, one arm-extensor exercise, and four to five additional exercises for the other main muscle groups. Exercising the major muscles will increase glucose uptake by increasing muscle mass.
- **Resistance bands** are an excellent alternative to weights for anyone who can't always get to the gym, needs a way to work out on vacation, or wants to create a home gym at a low cost.
- The standing poses found in **hatha yoga** use the weight of the body to develop resistance. Some poses proven to help with type 2 diabetes include the triangle, revolved triangle, plow, boat, supported bridge, supported shoulder stand, sideways angle, chair twist, downward-facing dog, and sun salutations.
- **Pilates** is a mindful training that includes a variety of exercises for core stability, muscular strength, flexibility, muscle control, posture, and breathing. It can be modified to include seated, standing, or lying

positions to protect the knee joints, avoid injury, and reduce blood sugar. Pilates equipment can accommodate many different body types. A Pilates program should include 5 minutes of warm-up exercises, 5 minutes of cool-down exercises, and 20 minutes of traditional Pilates exercises. A Pilates studio will offer mat classes or a variety of equipment, such as a Reformer, Cadillac, chair with adjustable spring resistance, or high barrel, as well as accessories such as magic circles and dumbbells.

Cardiovascular Exercise
Options:

- Aerobics
- Cycling
- Dance
- Jogging
- Cross-country skiing
- Hiking
- Mountain biking
- Rowing
- In-line skating
- Swimming

Swimming, in particular, provides an excellent workout for pitta people. It cools down pitta's heat and relaxes the mind. Swimming is an activity anyone can take up at any stage in life. The initial expense is low—all you need is a swimsuit. In the summer, it allows you to burn calories without getting overheated. In the colder months, indoor swimming can get you out of the house and keep you active.

Swimming has many health benefits. It is great for type 2 diabetes and weight management. It helps build strength, as it engages the arms, legs, and other major muscles of the body. It reduces blood pressure and cholesterol, minimizing the risk of stroke, heart attack, and type 2 diabetes. The breathing patterns used while swimming benefit lung health. The rhythmic breathing and calculated physical movements create a soothing sensation in both the mind and body.

Swimming is especially valuable for people with painful joints, as the buoyancy of the water takes pressure off the joints. Swimming poses a low risk of injury compared to many other cardio activities. Some people who are recovering from surgery can use swimming and regular pool workouts to ward off muscular atrophy.

If you are new to swimming, I suggest taking some adult swimming lessons. If you already know how to swim, start slowly and don't overdo it. Begin with a smooth, slow pace for no more than 15 or 20 minutes three times a week. Make a habit of monitoring your heart rate. Keep your leg kicks gentle to conserve energy. If you feel tired, switch to low-intensity strokes or use a kickboard.

No matter what exercises you choose to include in your 12-week program, start by making slow changes that will last. For some, that may mean walking for 5 minutes after each meal for the first week and then increasing to 10 minutes the next week. Do what works best for you and your body type, but be consistent in your practice. Don't procrastinate!

It's a good idea to plan your week and log your workouts so that you can keep track of your goals. Use the chart below, an app, or whatever you need to stay on top of your exercise. The chart below includes a column for each walk, resistance-training session, and cardio workout per week. Check off each column as you complete the exercise. A consistent exercise routine is crucial for the success of the program.

Exercise Journal

	10 min. walk	10 min. walk	10 min. walk	30 min. resistance	30 min. resistance	30 min. resistance	30 min. resistance
Week 1							
Week 2							
Week 3							
Week 4							
Week 5							
Week 6							
Week 7							
Week 8							
Week 9							
Week 10							
Week 11							
Week 12							

8-Week Supplement Schedule

See the Resources section at the back of this book for recommendations on where to purchase your herbs.

1. Barley tea

I recommend that everyone consume this daily. Look for hulled barley (also called Scotch barley) because unlike hull-less or pearl barley, it retains the bran, which delivers fiber in the form of complex carbohydrates.

Makes: about 3 cups

Ingredients:

- 3 cups hot water
- 2 tablespoons hulled barley
- 2 tablespoons almond milk
- ¼ teaspoon ground cinnamon
- ¼ teaspoon ground fenugreek
- ¼ teaspoon ground ginger
- ⅛ teaspoon ground turmeric
- a pinch of black pepper

Instructions: Bring the water to a boil in a saucepan over medium-high heat. Stir in barley, milk, cinnamon, fenugreek, ginger, turmeric, and pepper. Cover and reduce heat to medium-low. Simmer for 3 minutes. Enjoy.

2. Triphala

Recommended if you experience weight gain, gas, bloating, acidic belching, heartburn, heaviness after meals, lethargy, thick coating on the tongue, or excess mucus

Dosage: 1 teaspoon at night

3. Bitter melon

Recommended if you experience indigestion, low levels of insulin, or high post-meal blood glucose

Dosage: If you weigh under 200 pounds, ¼ teaspoon after breakfast and dinner. If you weigh over 200 pounds, ½ teaspoon after breakfast and dinner.

4. Gymnema sylvestre

Recommended if you experience sugar cravings, carbohydrate cravings, overeating, excessive appetite, sluggish digestion, or weight gain

Dosage: If you weigh under 200 pounds, ¼ teaspoon before breakfast and dinner. If you weigh over 200 pounds, ½ teaspoon before breakfast and dinner.

5. Neem

Recommended if you experience a high level of stress, inflammation in the digestive system, hyperacidity, ulcers, ulcerative colitis, Crohn's disease, or bowel congestion

Dosage: If you weigh under 200 pounds, ¼ teaspoon before breakfast and dinner. If you weigh over 200 pounds, ½ teaspoon before breakfast and dinner.

The 12-Week Program: 8-Week Constitution and Elimination Diet for Kapha

The goals for the 8-week constitution and elimination diet for kapha include reducing dense, sweet, salty, and sour foods that increase kapha, as well as including more pungent, bitter, and astringent foods. The sweet taste is found in sugary foods, starchy vegetables, certain fruits, and grains. White rice, white-flour products, other processed grains, ripe bananas, dates, and figs are all sweet. The salty taste is, of course, in salt. To reduce your intake of salt, cook at home, use whole ingredients, and avoid adding salt to foods. Restaurant food, canned goods, boxed foods, and processed foods are often heavily salted. Always read the nutritional-facts panel to determine the portion size and the amount of sodium. Packaged food items may include several small servings in one bag or box, so if you consume the entire package, you may consume several servings. This can make the total intake of sodium very high.

Pungent, bitter, and astringent are the best tastes for a kapha person. Pungent warms and flushes excess fluids and kapha secretions from the body. The pungent taste is often found in spicy, arid, and aromatic foods and herbs. The pungent taste purifies the blood, assists with weight loss, and has stimulating, sweat-inducing, and mucus-loosening actions. It improves metabolism, helps digestion, relieves congestion, promotes circulation, increases body temperature, and kills parasites. The pungent taste comes from aromatic oils commonly found in hot peppers, ginger, onion, radish, and other warming ingredients.

Bitter is the lightest and coolest of all the tastes. It purifies and dries up secretions, toning the body by reducing excess moisture. The bitter taste is often associated with reducing inflammation and fever. Bitter is detoxifying and antibacterial, so it is therefore used to cleanse the blood, reduce tumors, and stimulate the liver. Examples of bitter foods include dandelion leaves, bitter greens, aloe vera juice, and bitter melon.

The astringent taste heals, purifies, and constricts all body parts. It tightens and tones the tissues of the body and reduces secretions. Astringent herbs and foods promote healing, alleviate diarrhea, and promote the absorption of fluids. Astringent is anti-inflammatory, antibiotic, antibacterial, and hemostatic (stops bleeding). Examples of astringent foods and herbs include raspberry leaves, pomegranate, dandelion leaves, green beans, cranberries, and leafy green vegetables.

Try to include pungent, bitter, and astringent tastes in every meal. One of the easiest ways to do that is by adding herbs and spices to your food. Cumin, coriander, fennel, turmeric, fenugreek, and ginger make a great combination. You can make a culinary spice blend and use it on all your meals to ensure you are getting pungent, bitter, and astringent tastes.

Adding leafy greens to meals is a great way to include the bitter taste. You can put sautéed bitter greens in an egg-white omelet. For lunch, sauté some spinach and serve it with a grilled chicken breast. Mix a handful of kale into your soup for dinner.

Kapha people may like to snack, but it's best to avoid snacking while on the program. Watch your portion sizes and avoid overeating. Eat at regular mealtimes. This will help regulate your digestion. Most of your calories should come from vegetables on the kapha food list. Your plate should have about 50 percent vegetables and fruits, 25 percent lean protein, and 25 percent complex carbohydrates and clean fats.

Kapha Food Lists

Fruits to enjoy (generally astringent fruits): apples, cranberries, cherries, grapefruit, grapes, jackfruit (ripe), lemons, limes, oranges, pomegranates, prunes, rhubarb

Fruits to avoid (mostly sweet and sour fruits): avocados, bananas, dates, figs, kiwi, mangos, melons, papaya, pineapple, plums, watermelon

Vegetables to enjoy (bitter and pungent vegetables): artichoke, asparagus, beets, beet greens, bell peppers, bitter melon, bok choy, broccoli, Brussels sprouts, burdock root, cabbage, carrots, cauliflower, celery, chili peppers, corn, daikon radish, dandelion greens, eggplant, fennel, garlic, green beans, jackfruit (unripe), horseradish, kale, kohlrabi, leafy greens, leeks, lettuce, mushrooms, mustard greens, okra, onions, peas, radishes, rutabaga, scallions, seaweed, spaghetti squash, spinach, sprouts, tomatoes, turnip greens, turnips, watercress, wheatgrass

Vegetables to enjoy in moderation: zucchini

Vegetables to avoid (sweet and juicy veggies): cucumbers, olives, parsnips, potatoes, pumpkin, summer squash, sweet potatoes, taro root

---

Grains to enjoy: amaranth, barley, brown rice, buckwheat, quinoa, wild rice, black rice, rye

Grains to avoid: quick oats, white rice, wheat

Legumes to enjoy: azuki beans, black beans, black-eyed peas, chickpeas (garbanzo beans), lentils (red and brown), lima beans, mung beans, mung dal, navy beans, peas, pinto beans, split peas, tempeh, tofu (served warm), pigeon peas

Legumes to avoid: black lentils, kidney beans, soybeans

Dairy to enjoy: ghee

Dairy to avoid: buttermilk, butter, cheese, and all other products made from animal's milk

---

Meat and eggs to enjoy: chicken (white meat), turkey (white meat), venison, eggs

Meats to avoid: beef, buffalo, chicken (dark meat), turkey (dark meat), duck, lamb, pork, seafood

Condiments to enjoy: horseradish, kimchi, mustard without vinegar, sauerkraut

Condiments to avoid: ketchup, mayonnaise, pickles, soy sauce, tamari, vinegar, tahini

---

Nuts to enjoy: None! (Sorry!)

Seeds to enjoy: chia, flax, pumpkin, sunflower

Seeds to avoid: sesame, popcorn

Oils to enjoy (organic, cold pressed): almond, ghee, flaxseed, sesame, sunflower

Oils to avoid: avocado, apricot, coconut, olive, primrose, safflower, sesame, soybean, walnut

---

Beverages to enjoy: unsweetened soft cider, barley tea, black tea, unsweetened chai, flaxseed milk, black coffee, unsweetened cranberry juice, unsweetened pomegranate juice, warm unsweetened soy milk

Beverages to avoid: beer, wine, carbonated drinks, coconut milk, coconut water, sour cherry juice, chocolate milk, cold dairy drinks, iced tea, iced drinks, orange juice, papaya juice, rice milk, acidic juices, tomato juice, V8® juice

---

Spices to enjoy: All spices are fine!

Herbs to enjoy: alfalfa, aloe vera, basil, blackberry, burdock, chamomile, chicory, cilantro, dandelion, fennel, fenugreek, ginseng, hibiscus, jasmine, juniper berry, kukicha, lavender, lemon balm, lemongrass, nettle, oregano, parsley, passionflower, peppermint, raspberry leaf, red clover, rosemary, sarsaparilla, sassafras, spearmint, strawberry leaf, thyme, wintergreen, yarrow, yerba mate

Herbs to avoid: licorice, marshmallow, rosehip, slippery elm

Sweeteners to enjoy in moderation: applesauce, honey

Sweeteners to avoid: all others

Recipes for Kapha

BASIC KAPHA RECIPES

ALOE BASIL MARGARITA

Aloe vera cleanses the body as it flushes toxins from the blood and old bile from the gallbladder. Grow or buy whole-leaf aloe vera and slice the leaf to extract the gel. Savor this drink on a sunny afternoon!

Makes: Four 8-ounce glasses

Ingredients:

- 4 cups water
- Juice of 1 lemon
- Juice of ½ lime
- 3 fresh basil leaves
- 1 teaspoon grated fresh ginger
- 2 teaspoons aloe gel

Instructions:

Combine water, lemon juice, lime juice, basil, ginger, and aloe vera gel in a blender. Process on high for 30 seconds or until liquefied.

SPINACH PESTO

Garlic is one of the dominant flavors in traditional Mediterranean pesto, which is made with fresh herbs. Basil is generally the key herb in pesto, but any combination of fresh herbs and leafy green vegetables can be used in this nutrient-rich sauce.

Makes: 2 cups

Ingredients:

- ¼ cup raw sunflower seeds
- 2 to 3 cloves garlic
- ½ ripe avocado

- 2 cups packed baby spinach or roughly chopped mature spinach
- ½ cup coarsely chopped fresh parsley
- 3 tablespoons freshly squeezed lime or lemon juice
- 2 to 3 tablespoons extra-virgin sunflower oil

Instructions:

1. Combine sunflower seeds and garlic in a food processor. Process for 30 seconds or until coarsely chopped.
2. Add avocado, spinach, and parsley to the food processor and sprinkle lemon or lime juice on top. With the motor running, slowly add 2 tablespoons of the oil through the funnel in the lid and process for about 1 minute, stopping to scrape down the sides and to check on the consistency of the pesto. For a smoother, thinner consistency, add the remaining oil.

FIRE-ROASTED MARINARA

To make a heartier sauce, include meatballs made from unripe jackfruit or white meat turkey. Serve over spiraled vegetables such as broccoli stems, burdock root, rutabaga, or zucchini.

Makes: 6 to 10 servings

Ingredients:

- 5 tomatoes, halved
- 1 medium yellow onion, halved
- 1 head roasted garlic (see page 76)
- 1 cup lightly packed basil leaves
- 1 tablespoon chopped fresh oregano
- 1 tablespoon fresh thyme leaves
- 2 tablespoons freshly squeezed lemon or lime juice

Instructions:

1. Preheat oven to broil and move a rack to the top position. Line a rimmed baking sheet with parchment paper.
2. Arrange tomato and onion halves in one layer, cut side down, on prepared baking sheet. Broil in preheated oven for 3 minutes. Turn using tongs and broil for 3 more minutes or until the edges are charred. Remove from oven and set aside to cool slightly.
3. Combine garlic, basil, oregano, and thyme in a blender. Add lemon juice and process for 20 seconds. Scrape tomatoes and onions and their juices into the blender and process for 30 seconds or until smooth.

GRILLED SALSA

This grilled salsa is fun and easy to make. Tomatoes are an ideal low-glycemic food high in an antioxidant called lycopene, which is known for many health benefits, including reduced risk of heart disease and cancer.

Makes: 6 to 10 servings

Ingredients:

- 5 large tomatoes
- 1 yellow onion
- 1 jalapeno pepper
- 1 cup chopped fresh cilantro
- ½ teaspoon ground coriander
- ½ teaspoon ground cumin
- ½ teaspoon ground fenugreek
- ¼ teaspoon ground turmeric
- Juice of 1 lime

Instructions:

1. Preheat grill to high.
2. Slice tomatoes, onion, and pepper in half lengthwise. Place, cut side up, on the grill and cook for 2 minutes each side or until charred around the edges.
3. Transfer vegetables to a blender. Add cilantro, coriander, cumin, fenugreek, and turmeric. Drizzle lime juice on top and process for 1 minute or until blended and smooth.

KAPHA BREAKFAST

ARTICHOKE AND SUNDRIED TOMATO SCRAMBLE

Eating artichokes is a great way to reduce post-meal blood sugar. Include artichokes in a variety of breakfast scrambles to keep yourself satiated and balanced until lunch.

Makes: 2 servings

Ingredients:

- 1 tablespoon ghee (see page 164) or extra-virgin sunflower oil
- ½ onion, chopped
- ½ cup chopped artichoke hearts
- ¼ cup chopped sundried tomatoes
- 4 eggs, beaten

Instructions:

1. Heat ghee in a skillet over medium-high heat. Add onion and cook, stirring frequently, for 5 minutes or until soft and translucent.
2. Stir in artichokes and sundried tomatoes and reduce heat to medium. Pour eggs over vegetables and cook, stirring frequently, for about 7 minutes or

until eggs are cooked.

BLUEBERRY POWER BARS

No gluten, no sugar, no dairy! Tasty and surprisingly filling, these bars will power you up with no controversial ingredients. Try other dried berries such as cranberry or goji in this easy recipe.

Makes: about 12 squares

Ingredients:
- 2 tablespoons chia seeds
- ½ cup water
- 2 cups chopped dried blueberries or other dried berries
- ½ cup raw sunflower seeds
- ¼ cup flax seeds

Instructions:
1. Preheat oven to 300° F. Line a baking sheet with parchment paper.
2. Combine chia seeds and water in a small bowl and set aside for 5 minutes or until thickened.
3. Combine blueberries, sunflower seeds, and flax seeds in a mixing bowl. Stir in chia mixture. Scrape onto prepared baking sheet and pat, using the back of a spoon, into a rough square that is about ½ inch thick.
4. Bake in preheated oven for 20 minutes or until light golden brown. Remove, set aside to cool, and cut into 1 ½- to 2-inch squares. Store in an airtight container in the refrigerator for 7 to 10 days.

AMARANTH BREAKFAST BOWL

Amaranth was considered the grain of the gods by the Inca—perhaps because it provides energy, fiber, and endurance, which may be due to its high protein content. Loaded with antioxidants and inflammation-reducing nutrients, amaranth is an excellent gluten-free grain for all body types.

Makes: 2 servings

Ingredients:
- ½ cup amaranth
- ¼ cup hulled barley
- 1 cup warm water
- ⅔ cup unsweetened flaxseed milk or water
- ½ teaspoon ground cinnamon
- ¼ cup raw pumpkin seeds
- fresh fruit

Instructions:

1. Combine amaranth and barley in a small bowl. Add enough water to cover the grains. Cover and refrigerate overnight or for up to 24 hours.
2. The next morning, drain and rinse the amaranth mixture. Pour into a small saucepan and add flaxseed milk and cinnamon. Bring to a boil over medium-high heat. Reduce heat to medium-low, cover, and simmer, stirring occasionally, for 20 to 25 minutes or until grains are cooked and mixture is thickened.
3. Spoon into bowls, and sprinkle pumpkin seeds on top. Serve warm with fruit.

FRUIT SALAD
Pomegranate seeds are exceptional for controlling type 2 diabetes. They are high in antioxidants that repair the pancreas and improve blood sugar. Try adding fresh pomegranate seeds to teas and salads.
Makes: 1 to 2 servings
Ingredients:
- 1 pomegranate
- 1 green apple, thinly sliced
- 8 blackberries
- 4 strawberries, halved or quartered
- grated fresh ginger to taste

Instructions:
Cut pomegranate in half and scoop out the seeds into a bowl. Add apple, blackberries, and strawberries. Sprinkle ginger on top and toss to mix.

QUICK AND EASY QUINOA BOWL
Quinoa is often called a "superfood" and is a healthy choice because it is loaded with protein, fiber, B vitamins, and minerals. It's easy to make this bowl to power-start your day.
Makes: 2 servings
Ingredients:
- ½ cup quinoa
- 1 cup water
- ¼ cup berries or halved grapes, or ½ apple, chopped
- 2 tablespoons raw pumpkin or sunflower seeds
- unsweetened flaxseed milk, optional, to taste

Instructions:
1. Rinse quinoa in a fine mesh strainer under cool water. Shake and drain.
2. Bring water to a boil in a small saucepan over medium-high heat. Stir in quinoa, lower heat to medium-low, and simmer for 12 to 15 minutes or

until all of the water is absorbed. Remove from heat, cover, and set aside to steam for 5 minutes.

3. Divide quinoa between two bowls and add berries and seeds to each bowl. Serve with flaxseed milk if desired.

KAPHA LUNCH

CHICKEN AND SAUTÉED BRUSSELS SPROUTS

Brussels sprouts are high in fiber, which suppresses the appetite, satiates the body, and regulates blood sugar, reducing the risk of type 2 diabetes.

Makes: 2 to 3 servings

Ingredients:
- 1 boneless, skinless chicken breast, coarsely chopped
- 1 tablespoon ghee (see page 164) or extra-virgin sunflower oil
- 1 cup Brussels sprouts, sliced in half
- ½ red bell pepper, chopped
- ¼ small onion, chopped
- juice of 1 lemon

Instructions:
1. Place chicken pieces in a small saucepan and cover with water. Bring water to a boil over medium-high heat. Cover the pan, lower the heat to medium-low, and simmer for 5 to 7 minutes or until the center of the chicken turns opaque and the internal temperature reaches 165° F. Drain in a colander, rinse with cool water, and set aside.
2. Heat ghee in a large skillet over medium-high heat. Add Brussels sprouts, pepper, and onion. Cook, stirring frequently, for 5 minutes or until onion is soft and translucent.
3. Remove from heat and transfer to a bowl. Add chicken and lemon juice and toss to mix.

CHICKEN FAJITA BOWL

Use wild rice or black rice, not white rice, in this dish. Wild and black rice have more fiber and reduce blood sugar spikes. Serve with grilled salsa (see page 132).

Makes: 2 to 3 servings

Ingredients:
- 1 large boneless, skinless chicken breast, cut into ½-inch strips
- 1 tablespoon fajita seasoning (store bought or see recipe below)
- 1 tablespoon ghee (see page 164) or extra-virgin sesame oil, divided
- 1 red pepper, sliced

- 1 yellow pepper, sliced
- 1 onion, halved and sliced ½ inch thick
- 1 clove garlic, minced
- 2 cups cooked wild rice (see headnote above)
- ¼ cup chopped fresh cilantro

Instructions:
1. Combine chicken and seasoning in a bowl and toss to coat chicken strips.
2. Heat 1 teaspoon of the ghee in a large skillet over medium heat. Add chicken, cover, reduce heat to medium-low, and cook for 5 to 7 minutes. Flip the chicken strips and stir in remaining ghee, peppers, onion, and garlic. Cover and cook for about 5 minutes or until peppers are crisp-tender and the chicken's internal temperature reaches 165° F.
3. To assemble, spoon rice into two or three serving bowls. Arrange chicken and vegetables over rice and garnish with cilantro.

FAJITA SEASONING

Makes: 2 tablespoons (recipe may be doubled or tripled)
Ingredients:
- 1 tablespoon chili powder
- 1 teaspoon ground cumin
- 1 teaspoon ground fenugreek
- 1 teaspoon ground turmeric

Instructions:
Combine all ingredients in a jar with a lid. Cover and shake well.

MUSHROOM BARLEY CHICKEN STEW

You can use any type of mushroom in this recipe. If you are not a fan of mushrooms, substitute broccoli, green beans, corn, or bok choy.
Makes: 6 servings
Ingredients:
- 2 cups water
- ½ chicken, bone-in, cut into 3 or 4 pieces
- 1 cup hulled barley
- 1 teaspoon kelp
- 1 onion, quartered
- 3 cups chopped mushrooms
- 1 teaspoon ground fenugreek
- ½ teaspoon ground turmeric

Instructions:

1. Combine water and chicken in a large slow cooker. Stir in barley, kelp, onion, mushrooms, fenugreek, and turmeric. Cover, set to low heat, and cook for 6 to 8 hours or until the internal temperature of a large piece of chicken reaches 165° F.
2. Lift out chicken and cool slightly. Remove skin and bones, cut meat into small pieces, and return to liquid before serving.

EGGPLANT AND TURKEY WITH PESTO

Eggplant counteracts the enzyme that converts starch into blood sugar, making it a very effective food for preventing type 2 diabetes complications. Try eggplant spiraled into noodles or cut into steaks and grilled or baked.

Makes: 4 servings

Ingredients:
- 1 tablespoon ghee (see page 164) or extra-virgin sesame oil
- 1 boneless, skinless turkey breast, coarsely chopped
- 1 onion, chopped
- 2 cups chopped broccoli
- 1 eggplant, cut into spirals
- ½ cup pesto (see page 75)

Instructions:
Heat ghee in a large skillet over medium-high heat. Add turkey and onion and cook, stirring constantly, for 4 minutes or until turkey is lightly browned. Stir in broccoli and eggplant and cook, stirring frequently, for about 6 minutes or until vegetables are crisp-tender and the internal temperature of the turkey reaches 165° F. Remove from heat and transfer to a bowl. Stir in pesto and serve.

BEET AND CARROT SPIRALS WITH ROASTED VEGETABLES

This dish really celebrates kapha vegetables. Try adding ¼ cup chopped fresh herbs such as rosemary, parsley, oregano, or thyme to the dish before serving.

Makes: 6 servings

Ingredients:
- 2 red bell peppers, cut into eighths
- 2 leeks, split, washed, and cut into 2-inch lengths
- 1 onion, quartered
- 1 cup broccoli florets
- 1 cup cauliflower florets
- 2 tablespoons melted ghee (see page 164) or extra-virgin sesame oil, divided
- 2 carrots, spiralized
- 2 beets, spiralized

Instructions:

1. Preheat oven to 375° F. Line one large or two medium rimmed baking sheets with parchment paper.
2. Toss together the peppers, leeks, onion, broccoli, and cauliflower in a bowl. Drizzle 1 tablespoon of ghee on top and toss to coat. Spread vegetables in one layer on prepared pan(s). Roast in preheated oven for 25 minutes. Stir and return to the oven for 10 minutes or until vegetables are crisp-tender and slightly charred around the edges.
3. After stirring the vegetables, bring a pot of water to a boil over high heat. Add carrot and beet spirals, cover, lower heat, and simmer for 4 minutes or until tender. Drain, rinse, and transfer to a large bowl. Toss with remaining ghee and roasted vegetables.

KAPHA DINNER

CAULIFLOWER RICE WITH LEMON, KALE, AND PARSLEY

Adding herbs to your meals will enliven your tastebuds! Parsley is a wonderful addition to this recipe. It tastes great, lowers blood glucose, and tones the liver.

Makes: 4 to 6 servings

Ingredients:

- 1 small head cauliflower
- 3 tablespoons ghee (see page 164) or extra-virgin sunflower oil
- ½ onion, chopped
- ½ teaspoon ground fenugreek
- ¼ teaspoon ground turmeric
- ½ cup chopped kale
- 2 teaspoons lemon zest
- 4 tablespoons chopped fresh parsley

Instructions:

1. Trim cauliflower and place florets in a food processor or blender (you may have to do this in batches). Pulse until chopped to the size of grains of rice. Pour into a bowl and set aside.
2. Heat ghee in a large frying pan over medium heat. Add onion, fenugreek, and turmeric, and cook, stirring constantly, for 4 minutes. Stir in cauliflower and kale and cook, stirring frequently, for 6 to 8 minutes or until cauliflower is crisp-tender. Add lemon zest and parsley and toss to mix.

MUNG BEAN PATTIES

Mung bean patties are full of protein and fiber. Try them in place of a burger, served with sautéed vegetables and a cup of soup.

Makes: 4 patties

Ingredients:

- 1 cup dried mung beans, well rinsed
- 3 cups water
- Pinch of hing/asafetida (see headnote page 79)
- 1 small onion, finely chopped
- 1 tablespoon finely chopped garlic
- ½ teaspoon ground turmeric
- ⅓ cup raw pumpkin seeds
- 2 eggs, beaten
- 1 tablespoon ghee (see page 164) or extra-virgin sunflower oil
- ½ cup Mint-Cilantro Chutney (see following recipe)

Instructions:

1. The night before, cover beans with water in a large pot. Stir in hing and set aside to soak for 8 hours. Drain in a colander and rinse well.
2. The next day, pulse the beans in a food processor or mash them to break them into smaller pieces, but leave some whole for texture. Transfer to a large bowl and add onion, garlic, turmeric, and pumpkin seeds. Mix well. Drizzle eggs on top and toss to mix well.
3. Lightly oil the palms of your hands. Form four patties, patting them between your palms and shaping the edges with your fingers.
4. Heat ghee in a large skillet over medium-high heat. Add patties and cook for 3 minutes or until browned. Flip and cook for 3 more minutes or until browned on the opposite side. Serve with Mint-Cilantro Chutney.

MINT-CILANTRO CHUTNEY

Makes: about ½ cup

Ingredients:

- ¼ cup coarsely chopped fresh cilantro
- ¼ cup coarsely chopped fresh mint
- 1 teaspoon freshly grated ginger
- juice of ½ lemon
- 1 green serrano pepper, chopped

Instructions:

Combine cilantro, mint, ginger, lemon juice, and hot pepper in a food processor or blender. Process for 1 minute or until smooth, adding just enough cold water to keep the blades moving, or more if you like your chutney thin.

KAPHA VEGETABLE MUNG BEAN POTS WITH SEED CRUST

The seed crust is crunchy and makes a tasty topping for this bean-and-vegetable stew. Be sure to use ovenproof ramekins or small bowls for this dish.

Makes: 4 servings

Ingredients:

Bean Pots

- 1 ½ cups water or vegetable stock
- ½ cup split dried mung beans, well rinsed
- 2 tablespoons ghee (see page 164), divided
- 1 onion, chopped
- 1 celery stalk, chopped
- 1 small zucchini, chopped
- 3 cloves garlic, finely chopped
- 1 cup tomato sauce, store-bought or Fire-Roasted Marinara (see page 132)

Seed Crust

- ½ cup cooked wild rice or black rice
- ¼ cup raw sunflower seeds
- 2 tablespoons raw pumpkin seeds
- 1 tablespoon flaxseeds
- about 3 tablespoons sunflower or almond oil

Instructions:

1. Bring water to a boil in a saucepan over high heat. Add beans, reduce heat to medium-high, and simmer for 30 minutes or until tender. Drain and combine with 1 tablespoon of ghee in a bowl. Set aside.

2. Preheat oven to 375° F. Place four heatproof ramekins on a baking sheet and set aside.

3. Meanwhile, heat remaining ghee in a large skillet over medium-high heat. Add onion and cook, stirring occasionally, for 5 minutes. Add celery, zucchini, and garlic and cook, stirring frequently, for 5 minutes or until vegetables are tender. Remove from heat and stir in tomato sauce and cooked mung beans. Spoon mixture into ramekins.

4. To make the seed crust, combine the rice and seeds in a food processor. With the motor running, add oil through the funnel in the lid until the mixture starts to clump together. Divide crust mixture into four equal portions and pat over vegetable mixture in ramekins. Bake in preheated oven for 30 minutes or until bean mixture is bubbling and crust is browned.

CAULIFLOWER FENNEL SOUP

Fennel bulbs and stems have a mild anise flavor that complements many cooked dishes, as well as salads.

Makes: 4 to 6 servings

Ingredients:

- 2 tablespoons ghee (see page 164)
- 1 teaspoon mustard seeds
- 4 stalks celery, chopped
- 1 medium yellow onion, chopped
- 2 fennel bulbs, chopped
- 3 leeks, washed and coarsely chopped
- 8 cups water
- 1 head cauliflower, roughly chopped
- ¼ cup chopped fresh dill
- 3 tablespoons chopped fresh parsley

Instructions:

1. Heat ghee in a large saucepan over medium-high heat. Add mustard seeds, cover, reduce heat to medium-low, and cook for 2 minutes or until all the seeds pop.
2. Stir in celery and onion and cook, stirring frequently, for 5 minutes. Add fennel and leeks and cook, stirring frequently, for 5 minutes. Add water and bring to a boil over high heat. Add cauliflower and cook for about 15 minutes or until tender.
3. Transfer vegetables and liquid to a blender in batches and process on high for 1 minute or until smooth. Pour back into the saucepan and heat through over medium-high heat, stirring constantly.

CHICKPEA VEGETABLE SOUP

Chickpeas, also called garbanzo beans, are a high-protein, high-fiber, low-glycemic legume. If using canned chickpeas, be sure there is no sodium added. To use dried chickpeas, soak them overnight in water with a pinch of hing (asafetida). The next day, drain, rinse well, and increase the boil time in step 2 to 40 minutes.

Makes: 4 to 6 servings

Ingredients:

- 1 tablespoon extra-virgin sunflower oil or ghee (see page 164)
- 1 small onion, chopped
- 1 clove garlic, chopped
- 1 cup chopped kale
- 2 ½ cups water
- 1 teaspoon dried oregano
- 1 cup fresh or frozen (thawed) peas

- 1 cup fresh or frozen (thawed) corn
- 1 can (15 ounces) chickpeas, drained and rinsed
- 2 tomatoes, chopped

Instructions:

1. In a large saucepan, heat oil over medium-high heat. Add onion and cook, stirring frequently, for 5 minutes or until translucent. Stir in garlic and kale and cook, stirring frequently, for 4 more minutes.
2. Add water, oregano, peas, corn, chickpeas, and tomatoes. Reduce heat to medium-low and simmer, stirring occasionally, for 10 minutes.

ROASTED GARLIC AND MUNG BEANS

The mung bean is a versatile bean that absorbs the flavors of the herbs and spices in this recipe. Soaking beans with a pinch of hing (asafetida) helps to prevent gas or indigestion. Serve with sautéed or steamed veggies.

Makes: 2 to 3 servings

Ingredients:

- 1 cup dried mung beans, well rinsed
- 3 cups water
- pinch of hing/asafetida (see headnote, page 79)
- 1 tablespoon ghee (see page 164)
- 2 to 4 cloves roasted garlic (see page 76)
- 1 teaspoon ground cumin
- ¼ teaspoon ground coriander
- ¼ teaspoon ground turmeric

Instructions:

1. The night before, cover beans with water in a large bowl. Stir in hing and set aside to soak.
2. The next day, drain beans in a colander and rinse well.
3. Heat ghee in a saucepan over medium-high heat. Stir in garlic, cumin, coriander, and turmeric. Break up garlic with the back of a wooden spoon and cook, stirring constantly, for 1 minute. Add beans and heat, stirring frequently, for 2 minutes or until warmed through.

Sleep Optimization

Kapha people usually do not have difficulty sleeping. However, because they have more heaviness in their constitution, they find it difficult to wake and get going in the morning. To feel less tired in the morning, eat a light, early dinner and do not snack after dinner. Eating earlier will give your body plenty of time to digest so that it can focus on detoxifying while you are sleeping. Once your body does not have the burden of digestion, it can work on cleaning the tissues and removing waste. This will reduce the heavy feeling you may have in the morning and allow you to wake up feeling refreshed.

Kapha people do not need as much sleep as vata or pitta people, so they can stay up a little later and get up earlier. Kapha people need to get out of bed before 6 a.m. and not oversleep. Kapha time is from 6 to 10 a.m., and the longer you stay in bed during that timeframe, the more you may experience feelings of lethargy and tiredness. Kapha is responsible for the structure and cohesiveness of the body. That means that if you are still in bed after 6 a.m., your body becomes stiff and heavy. If you are up, moving around, and exercising, the kapha energy will help your body build muscle. Your lungs are at their strongest during the kapha time of day, so you will receive the most benefits from exercise during the 6 to 10 a.m. kapha window.

Kapha Daily Schedule
Wake up: 4:00–5:00 a.m.
30 minute exercise
Breakfast: 6:30–7:30 a.m.
15-minute walk
Lunch: 12:30–1:30 p.m.
15-minute walk
Dinner: 5:30–6:30 p.m.
15-minute walk
30-minute relaxation
Go to sleep: 9:30–10:30 p.m.

Lifestyle Enhancement
Kapha people naturally have more heaviness in the mind and body. To keep kapha balanced, include activities that are engaging and keep you active, moving, and challenged. Kapha people also tend to have more difficulty staying motivated. The kapha lifestyle-enhancement program therefore includes group support and motivational strategies to help you stay committed. Kapha people are often content to just relax and hang out, so they must continually work toward reducing sedentary behaviors. They need to get up and move regularly. Regular movement will help them stay balanced. Do not stay seated for too long. Break up sedentary activities such as watching TV, using the computer, or reading by doing chores around the house, taking a quick walk, or stretching. Do not overeat or oversleep. Stay engaged with the world both mentally and physically,

and you will feel your best!

Techniques to Balance the Kapha Mind and Body
- Engage in regular and vigorous group exercises.
- Break a sweat when working out.
- Wake up early and get moving.
- Avoid cold and damp environments.
- Drink warming herbal teas and fluids.
- Use self-motivational therapies.
- Eat warm vegetable soups.
- Avoid sitting for long periods.

30-Minute Daily Relaxation Practice
Allow 30 minutes for your relaxation practice, which includes restorative yoga poses, breathwork, and meditation. If you are new to these practices, don't be afraid to give them a try. The yoga poses are gentle and relaxing. Yoga has been shown to improve sleep length and quality. The recommended breathwork is soothing, and you may notice an immediate effect on stress reduction. The meditation is a simple exercise that you can do on your own or with guided audio.

Try to do your relaxation practice every day. Aim for 30 minutes, but if you can't get 30 minutes in, please do any amount you can. A little is better than nothing, and consistency is more beneficial than irregularity. Once you begin to explore your relaxation practice, you may find that you gravitate toward one activity over another. If that happens, feel free to alter the amount of time spent in each activity. I recommend setting a timer so you can fully relax and not watch the clock.

20-Minute Yoga Practice
Start with a loosening practice. While standing, draw figure eights in the air with your nose to release neck tension. Draw several figure eights horizontally and vertically. Then work on rotating your joints. Rotate your shoulders, elbows, wrists, hips, knees, and ankles. Rotate clockwise and counterclockwise several times.

Kneeling Forward Bend (Mandukasana)
Duration: 3 to 4 minutes
Benefits: Tones the organs; stimulates the pancreas; relieves constipation; reduces belly fat; improves digestive function; stretches the back; alleviates pain in the legs, knees, and ankles
Contraindications: back pain, knee pain, pregnancy

Instructions: Start by sitting in a kneeling position. If it is uncomfortable to kneel, sit in a chair. Make fists with your thumb tucked inside your four fingers with both hands. Place your fists on the abdomen on either side of your navel, take a deep inhale, and elongate your spine. On the exhale, contract your abdomen inward, and slowly bend forward, pressing your fists into your abdomen. Keep your spine and neck long; do not slouch. Keep your gaze looking forward. Hold the pose, slowly inhaling and exhaling. When you are ready to release, inhale and slowly raise your trunk, relaxing your hands. Repeat this process four or five times.

Seated Spinal Twist *(Vakrasana)*

Duration: 3 to 4 minutes

Benefits: Massages the abdominal organs, improves digestion, reduces constipation, reduces belly fat, relieves vertebral stiffness

Contraindications: Ulcers; slipped disc; severe spine, shoulder, or hip injury

Instructions: Sit on the floor with a straight spine and your legs extended in front of you. On an inhale, bend your right knee upward and place your right foot flat on the floor next to your left thigh. Exhale, turn toward your right knee, wrap your left arm around your right knee, and simultaneously place your right hand behind your right buttock on the floor. Use your right arm to sit up straight and support the spine. Stay here for five breaths or more. Exit the pose on an inhale, release your left arm from your knee, and release the twist so you are facing forward. Exhale, straightening your right knee. Repeat on the opposite side, with your left knee bent and your right arm clasping your left knee. Put your left hand behind your left buttock for support.

Extended-Leg Forward Bend *(Paschimatanasana)*

Duration: 3 to 4 minutes

Benefits: Calms the mind, reduces stress and anxiety, stimulates the liver, improves digestion

Contraindications: Slipped disc

Instructions: Sit on the floor with your legs straight in front of you. Press actively through your heels and flex your feet. Gently press your thighs into the floor. Place your hands on the floor beside your hips. Keep your chest lifted. Exhale and lean forward from your hip joints, not your waist. Lengthen your tailbone away from the back of your pelvis. Let your arms reach toward your feet and let them rest on your legs without straining yourself. With each inhalation, lift and lengthen your torso slightly; with each exhalation, release a little deeper into the forward bend. Stay in the pose anywhere from 1 to 3 minutes. To release the pose, exhale and lift your torso away from your thighs.

Cobra Pose *(Bhujangasana)*
Duration: 3 to 4 minutes
Benefits: Relieves stress, opens the lungs, stimulates abdominal organs, strengthens the spine
Contraindications: spondylitis (a type of arthritis of the spine), back or neck pain
Instructions: Lie on your stomach, toes pointing straight back, hands underneath your shoulders, and elbows close to your body. Keep your legs engaged and glutes relaxed. On an inhale, lift your chest. Pull your shoulder blades together and slightly down the spine. Lift your head last. Gently press into your hands, opening your chest. Extend out through the toes. Come down on an exhale. Repeat several times.

Corpse Pose *(Savasana)*
Duration: 3 to 4 minutes
Benefits: Calms the mind; relieves stress and mild depression; relaxes the body; alleviates headaches, fatigue, and insomnia; lowers blood pressure
Contraindications: None known
Instructions:
- For this pose you will need two rolled-up towels, pillows, or blankets.
- To begin, sit on the floor with your knees bent, feet on the floor, and lean back onto your forearms and come all the way down to a lying position.
- Place one rolled-up towel under your knees and the other under your neck.
- Inhale and slowly extend the right leg, then the left, pushing through the heels. Release both legs, softening into the groin. Try to keep the legs angled evenly to the midline of the torso, and let the feet turn out equally.
- Reach your arms toward the ceiling, perpendicular to the floor. Rock slightly from side to side and broaden the back ribs and the shoulder blades away from the spine. Then release the arms to the floor. Rest the backs of the hands on the floor several inches away from your body.
- Soften your face, eyes, and tongue. Let your eyes sink deeply into the sockets.
- Make any final adjustments you need, and then relax and allow yourself to become still.

5-Minute Breathwork: Breath of Fire *(Kapal Bhati)*

Benefits: Enhances the insulin receptors in muscles and increases glucose uptake by cells, reducing blood sugar

Contraindications: Lung disease

Instructions:

- Find a comfortable, upright, seated position.
- Place your hands on your belly and, on an inhale, feel it expand out and then, on an exhale, gently pull back.
- Exhale through both nostrils, firmly contracting the belly toward the spine.
- Inhale. The inhale should be natural, light, and through both nostrils.
- Continue to be aware of your exhales and inhales. The breath should be in the abdomen with an emphasis on the exhale, letting the inhale come as a natural reflex.
- Feel the rhythmic cycles of the breath and the pumping action of the abdomen.
- Duration: After one series of breaths, lasting no longer than one minute, rest and breathe naturally. Then repeat. Begin with three rounds and increase over time.

5-Minute Awareness Meditation

An awareness meditation is a mindfulness practice that allows us to become aware of our thoughts and environment. It brings light to the storylines we create in our mind and the sounds and smells present in our environment. Through awareness meditation, we can train our brain to notice our mental habits—the good and the bad—and by noticing these habits, we can change our self-limiting beliefs and negative thought patterns.

Awareness meditation is also great for improving concentration and focus. It helps us stay more alert, because we quickly become aware of distracting thoughts. The sooner we become aware of these distractions, the sooner we can bring our attention back to the area of focus.

AWARENESS MEDITATION PRACTICE

1. Start by finding a comfortable seated position. Sit with your spine straight but not rigid; it's a position of ease. You can sit in a chair or on the floor, whichever is more comfortable for you. Allow your body to become still. Either soften your gaze and look toward your nose or close your eyes.

2. To settle in, take a few deep belly breaths. As you inhale through your nostrils, let your belly expand outward and, on the exhale, allow your belly to

gently contract inward. Check in with your body. Notice any tension or tightness. Are there any emotions associated with the tension? Do you feel anxiousness or calm? What's going on in your mind? Are there a lot of busy thoughts, or are you calm and content?

3. Notice your breath. Feel your inhalation, the pause. Feel the exhalation, the pause. Rest your awareness on the pauses between the breaths.

4. If at any point your mind wanders, notice the thought without judgment. You may want to label the thought as "past," "present," or "future"—something simple to acknowledge the thought without an emotion—and then bring your attention back to the breath. Thoughts are like cars on a road; you simply watch them pass by and don't jump into the car. If a thought carries you away, gently bring your attention back to the breath. Spend a couple of minutes observing your thoughts.

5. Next, expand your awareness outside your body to the sounds around you. Take a moment to notice the rise and fall of sounds. Whenever your mind wanders, gently go back to sounds. Spend a few minutes here.

6. Gently come back to the breath. Notice how your body expands on an inhalation and contracts on an exhalation. Thank yourself for taking time to engage in a mindful practice that will benefit your health and well-being.

It's a good idea to keep a daily log of your relaxation practice. This way, you can check off the days and remember to include it in your schedule. You may also want to note any feelings or sensations that arise during your practice. Remember that it *is* a practice; the first days are the hardest days, and they may feel awkward. But it gets more comfortable, I promise!

DAILY RELAXATION JOURNAL

	Sunday	Monday	Tuesday	Wednesday	Thursday	Friday	Saturday
Week 1							
Week 2							
Week 3							
Week 4							
Week 5							
Week 6							
Week 7							
Week 8							
Week 9							
Week 10							
Week 11							
Week 12							

Weekly Exercise

The kapha person naturally has a thicker, sturdier body structure and lots of endurance. Having a stout form can put extra stress on the joints, so be mindful of any activity that irritates your knees, hips, or ankles. The kapha exercise program includes a little bit of everything: regular walking, cardio workouts, and resistance training. Kapha people can gravitate toward stagnation, so it's important to include movement to stay balanced. Kapha people must sweat and engage in challenging exercises. According to Ayurveda, sweat is a byproduct of fat tissue, so through sweating, we purify fat. The kapha person naturally has a slow and steady pace, so it's a good idea to include bursts of energy to help you break into a sweat.

For a kapha person, it is essential to stay engaged. Having an exercise partner or a personal trainer will help you stay motivated. Team sports are great for kapha people. They get motivational support from others, and they must commit to a schedule.

There are many different forms of exercise you can use for resistance and cardio workouts. It's important to do activities that you enjoy—I can't stress that enough. Examples of resistance training include weightlifting, hatha yoga, and Pilates. Cardio workouts include activities such as vinyasa yoga, dance, aerobics, and jogging. There are a few activities that are especially beneficial for kapha people: interval workouts, fartlek, hill repeats, cycling, boot camp, and hot or flow types of yoga.

If you are new to exercising, start by making slow changes that will last. For some, that may mean walking for 5 minutes after each meal and increasing to 15 minutes the second week and adding resistance training the third week. Do what works best for you so that you can continue the practice long after the 12-week program. But don't procrastinate!

WEEKLY EXERCISE PROGRAM

- 150 minutes of weekly exercise
  - 30 minutes of resistance training twice a week
  - 30 minutes of cardiovascular exercise three times a week

- 45 minutes of daily walking
  - Three 15-minute walks after meals or 45 minutes daily

Interval Workouts

Interval workouts alternate between two sets. The first set is a burst into a faster-paced walk or run, and the second set is a slower-paced recovery walk or jog.

There are three basic types of interval workouts:

1. **Repeats**: The fast-pace distance is equal to the recovery distance. *Example:* Run one block and walk one block.
2. **Ladders**: The length of the intervals either steadily increases or decreases. *Example:* Run two blocks, walk two blocks, run one block, walk one block, run a half block, walk a half block. *In reverse:* Run a half block, walk a half block, run one block, walk one block, run two blocks, walk two blocks.
3. **Pyramids**: The length of the intervals peaks and then returns to the beginning length. *Example:* Run 220 meters, then 440 meters, then 880 meters, then back to 440 meters, then 220 meters again. Pyramids should be done on a track with defined distances to be more accurate. Always do a recovery walk following each running interval. The walking distance should be at least half your running distance, but can be more depending on your experience.

Fartlek

Fartlek is a silly-sounding Swedish term meaning "speed play." Fartlek is a less structured type of interval training where you add bursts of speed at various times during your walk or run. Fartlek training prepares your legs to experience a variety of paces and increases your awareness of your ability to maintain fluctuating rhythms at various distances. Fartlek can be part of your daily walks. A fartlek run consists of an easy-paced warm-up walk or jog, a burst of speed into a run or jog, and a recovery. Speed bursts should last from 15 seconds up to 3 minutes, while recovery time should be about two-thirds of the burst time.

Hill Repeats

Hill repeats are quick-paced uphill walks or jogs used for strength and cardio training. If you have hills in your neighborhood, this is a great place to start. Walking or running uphill lessens the impact force, thus reducing possible overuse injuries. Once at the top of the hill, you can walk or jog slowly back to the bottom of the hill and then repeat the uphill.

Cycling

Cycling is a cardio exercise with many health benefits. Kids and adults of all ages can enjoy a great workout—and have fun along the way. Cycling improves overall balance and coordination and increases your metabolism to help you burn more calories and shed excess weight. It is an excellent activity for kapha people because it can be done with others as a motivational group bike ride. Through cycling, you can explore and discover new trails and places in nature.

Cycling is also a great way to commute to work. Instead of the stress and anxiety of sitting in traffic, you can enjoy the pleasure and satisfaction of riding a bike.

Cycling reduces the risk of heart disease. It causes you to breathe deeper and sweat, both of which are very beneficial for kapha. Cycling takes impact off the joints, allowing the lower body to get a workout without the stress and impact of additional weight on the joints. As you continue to cycle, you will gain more stamina and energy for your daily activities.

Before starting a cycling program, get properly outfitted and versed in correct posture and technique. New cyclists should begin with a half-hour ride every other day. Take it slow and easy at first. If you can do it without getting out of breath, you can slowly increase the amount of time. Choose one day a week to push yourself on hills. You should always warm up properly and have a rest day after a long bike ride. Soon you will start to notice your rides getting smoother and longer, and you will feel more energetic with less recovery time.

Boot Camp

Boot-camp workouts are intense, calorie-burning workouts that are great for weight loss. Boot camp is excellent for kapha people because the social interactions will keep you motivated and engaged. Workouts are much more fun with others who have similar goals and fitness levels. Social support creates a bond that will keep you coming back for more.

Boot camps involve moving through various stations that improve mobility skills, balance, strength, and coordination. Many of the exercises use body weight for resistance training. The combination of cardiovascular and resistance training leads to incredible definition and muscle tone. Here are some examples of boot-camp exercises:

- **Suicide Runs**: Set up four different cones on a field at various distances. Run to the first cone, touch it, and then run back to the beginning. Run to the second cone and touch it, and then run back to the start once again. Continue the same procedure for the third and fourth cones, take a rest, and repeat from the beginning.
- **Box Jumps:** Place some form of a box or high step directly in front of you. Then squat down and jump with both legs onto the box. Jump back down to complete a rep, and then do another one, shooting for a total of 10 reps. The higher the box, the more difficult it gets!
- **Push-Up-Squat-Crunch Circuit**: This is simpler than it sounds. Perform as many push-ups as you can in one minute, then as many squats as you can in one minute, and finally as many crunches as you can in one minute. This is an excellent exercise for targeting all the main muscle

groups and increasing overall body strength.

- **Farmer's Carry**: Pick up a heavy object such as a dumbbell and walk across a field with it. The farmer's carry increases grip, core, leg, and shoulder strength.

There are many more boot-camp exercises, and you can create some of your own after a little experience in class. There are a variety of camps out there, so find one that suits you. If you want to get in better shape, burn some calories, and make some new friends in the process, boot camp is a great option!

Yoga

More active types of yoga, such as flow classes and hot yoga, can provide excellent cardio and resistance training. Yoga can tone and condition the body while calming and balancing the mind for complete physical, mental, and spiritual health.

The health benefits of a regular yoga practice include relief of back, neck, and joint pain; release of shoulder tension; superb toning and flexibility of the whole body; strengthening of all the muscles, tendons, and ligaments; and improved posture. The discipline and awareness required to maintain the alignment of the postures can also help you maintain correct posture in your daily activities and prevent chronic injuries.

Hot yoga is detoxifying, as sweating releases water-soluble toxins from the body. Flow-type yoga classes coordinate breath with movement. The Surya Namaskar, or sun salutation, flow series has nine movements with inhalations and exhalations corresponding to each movement. It is an excellent mindful aerobic exercise that helps balance kapha and reduce blood sugar.

Other Cardio Options

- Aerobics
- Baseball
- Badminton
- Basketball
- Bowling
- Dance
- Cross-country skiing
- Football
- Kayaking
- Racquetball
- Martial arts
- Mountain biking
- Pickleball
- Roller skating/blading
- Soccer
- Stair stepping
- Swimming
- Tennis

Whatever activities you choose, always make your exercise program fun, and you can be confident that it will help you manage your blood sugar and weight.

It's a good idea to plan your week and log your workouts so that you can keep track of your goals. Use the chart below, an app, or whatever you need to stay on top of your exercise. The chart below includes a column for each walk, resistance-training session, and cardio exercise per week. Please check off each column as you complete the exercise. A consistent exercise routine is crucial for the success of the program.

Exercise Journal

	15 min. walk	15 min. walk	15 min. walk	30 min. cardio	30 min. cardio	30 min. cardio	30 min. resistance	30 min. resistance
Week 1								
Week 2								
Week 3								
Week 4								
Week 5								
Week 6								
Week 7								
Week 8								
Week 9								
Week 10								
Week 11								
Week 12								

8-Week Supplement Schedule

See the Resources section at the back of this book for recommendations on where to purchase your herbs.

1. Barley tea

I recommend that everyone consume this daily. Look for hulled barley (also called Scotch barley) because unlike hull-less or pearl barley, it retains the bran, which delivers fiber in the form of complex carbohydrates.

Makes: about 3 cups
Ingredients:
- 3 cups hot water

- 2 tablespoons hulled barley
- 2 tablespoons almond milk
- ¼ teaspoon ground cinnamon
- ¼ teaspoon ground fenugreek
- ¼ teaspoon ground ginger
- ⅛ teaspoon ground turmeric
- a pinch of black pepper

Instructions: Bring the water to a boil in a saucepan over medium-high heat. Stir in barley, milk, cinnamon, fenugreek, ginger, turmeric, and pepper. Cover and reduce heat to medium-low. Simmer for 3 minutes. Enjoy.

2. Triphala

Recommended if you experience weight gain, sluggish bowel movements, heaviness after meals, lethargy, thick coating on the tongue, or excess mucus

Dosage: 1 teaspoon at night

3. Bitter melon

Recommended if you experience indigestion, low levels of insulin, or high post-meal blood glucose

Dosage: If you weigh under 200 pounds, ¼ teaspoon after breakfast and dinner. If you weigh over 200 pounds, ½ teaspoon after breakfast and dinner.

4. Tulsi

Recommended if you experience low energy, fatigue, inflammation, pain, swelling, gas and bloating, weight gain, brain fog, or mood swings

Dosage: If you weigh under 200 pounds, ¼ teaspoon before breakfast and dinner.

If you weigh over 200 pounds, ½ teaspoon before breakfast and dinner.

5. Gymnema sylvestre

Recommended if you experience sugar cravings, carbohydrate cravings, overeating, excessive appetite, sluggish digestion, or weight gain

Dosage: If you weigh under 200 pounds, ¼ teaspoon before breakfast and dinner. If you weigh over 200 pounds, ½ teaspoon before breakfast and dinner.

6. Neem

Recommended if you experience a high level of stress, inflammation in the digestive system, hyperacidity, ulcers, ulcerative colitis, Crohn's disease, or bowel congestion

Dosage: If you weigh under 200 pounds, ¼ teaspoon before breakfast and dinner. If you weigh over 200 pounds, ½ teaspoon before breakfast and dinner.

CHAPTER 9

The 12-Week Program: 1-Week Detox and Restoration

Congratulations! You made it through the 8-week constitution and elimination diet. Completing this is not an easy feat, so give yourself a warm pat on the back. Diet and lifestyle habits are hard to break. But as you integrated new foods and a balancing routine into your life, I'm sure you noticed a positive change that kept you motivated. You improved your energy, physical symptoms, elimination, digestion, and mental well-being during the 8 weeks. The tea, dietary choices, and regular mealtimes all improved your digestive fire and metabolism. The daily exercise strengthened your body and increased your muscle mass, promoting glucose uptake. The relaxation practice calmed your mind, easing stress-induced spikes in blood sugar. The regular sleep schedule helped regulate your body's natural rhythms. And the supplements worked hard to manage blood glucose and reduce your symptoms. Once you start to feel good, it's easy to continue on the path to wellness. Seasonal detoxification is part of the Ayurvedic lifestyle, so our next stop is the detoxification and restoration week.

Reasons to Detoxify

Unfortunately, we live in a very toxic world. The air we breathe is polluted, the water we drink is contaminated, and much of the food we eat is highly processed. Trying to live a wholesome, healthy lifestyle now is more challenging than ever before, making seasonal detoxification a must.

The standard Western diet contributes to poor health because it lacks the nutrients and fiber our bodies need. What, how, and when we eat are all factors that contribute to the development of metabolic waste. When we eat under stress or eat foods that are heavy, sweet, or greasy, our digestive fire diminishes, and we cannot break down and assimilate food. Undigested food turns into metabolic waste, and, as this waste builds in the body, it interferes with the body's natural functions.

The average Western diet consists of high-sugar, low-fiber, and refined foods, including white flour, processed meat, saturated fat, alcohol, preservatives, and additives. This type of diet does not include the amount of fiber needed to eliminate toxins from the body. A poor-quality diet that lacks fiber causes stagnation in the colon; to have a well-functioning immune system, the colon must be clean. An easy way to check the health of your colon is to look at your tongue. Your tongue is a reflection of your digestive system. The area close to the tip of the tongue represents the upper part of the digestive system and the back of the tongue represents the colon. If you have a thick coating on the back of your tongue, you have metabolic waste in your colon.

Toxicity forms in an unhealthy large intestine, or colon. The colon is approximately 5 to 5 1/2 feet long and 2 1/2 inches in diameter and makes up the end portion of the digestive tract. It contains nearly 60 varieties of microflora or bacteria that aid in digestion, promote vital nutrient production, maintain pH (acidic-alkaline) balance, and prevent the proliferation of harmful bacteria. The beneficial bacteria provide essential functions such as the synthesis of folic acid and valuable nutrients from foods, including vitamin K and some B vitamins.

In a healthy colon, the beneficial bacteria make up at least 85 percent of the population, and the harmful bacteria comprise 15 percent or less. However, a diet high in simple carbs and sugar feeds the harmful bacteria. The harmful bacteria multiply in the colon and can migrate into the bloodstream and small intestine, where they can cause further injury in the digestive system and throughout the body.

Recognizing Toxicity

Constipation, mucus, and bloody stools are common signs of colon toxicity. Last year, Americans spent over $1.4 billion on over-the-counter laxatives. We have a problem with constipation! Constipation occurs from a lack of fiber and consuming too many dry and processed foods. This causes the colon to become dry and fecal matter hard and sticky. Bowel movements are infrequent and incomplete, causing difficulty and straining; and the stools become hardened pebbles. The dry, impacted colon then becomes inflamed. The body responds by producing mucus to lubricate the inflamed tissues. Elimination then changes from hard, dry stools to stools with mucus or loose stools. The accumulation of mucus, inflammation, and hardened feces results in a much narrower stool— sometimes even as thin as a pencil.

A person with a healthy colon should have a daily bowel movement. Elimination should be in the morning, complete and smooth, and without straining, blood, or mucus. The stool should be light brown in color, well-formed, and shaped like a banana. There should be little or no offensive odor, and the stool should not stick to the toilet after flushing. Having infrequent, hard, sinking, loose, or sticky stools or stools with mucus or blood is indicative of a problem. Another telltale sign of toxicity is the classic "potbelly." A person can't have a flat abdomen if they are carrying waste. Even thin people can have protruding stomachs. Feeling gassy, bloated, and heavy are all problems related to toxicity.

Many people become accustomed to feeling toxic, tired, bloated, constipated, inflamed, mentally sluggish, or overweight. Eventually, this becomes a way of life, and they don't suspect they have a health issue. They may use medications to cover up the symptoms, but they never correct the underlying cause. Toxicity can contribute to many common health problems, such as the following:

- Allergies
- Arthritis
- Asthma
- Backaches
- Bad breath/halitosis
- Chronic fatigue
- Constipation
- Depression
- Distended abdomen
- Foul body odor
- Frequent colds
- Gas
- Headaches
- Hemorrhoids
- Hypertension
- Indigestion
- Insomnia
- Irritability
- Loose stools
- Menstrual problems
- Skin problems
- Weight gain

Chronic toxicity can also lead to the following more severe conditions:

1. **Bowel toxemia**: This is a condition caused by years of waste material, impacted feces, bacteria, fungi, viruses, dead cellular tissue, and accumulated mucus in the colon. This condition can inhibit muscular action, causing sluggish bowel movements, constipation, and inflammation.

2. **Gut permeability**: Over time, tiny cracks develop in the intestinal wall, and undigested foods and metabolic waste permeate through the intestinal wall and into the bloodstream. These toxins can impair healthy liver, lung, and kidney function. A person with this condition will have food sensitivities and feel tired or ill frequently.

3. **Parasites**: Metabolic waste is the perfect breeding ground for parasites. The most common sources of parasitic infections are undercooked meats (beef, pork, and raw fish, especially), unwashed fruits and vegetables, travel to third-world countries, contaminated water, mosquitoes, and pets. Humans play host to thousands of different kinds of bacteria and other

microorganisms. Most of these reside in the colon, but they can migrate to other parts of the body, including the liver, lungs, muscles, joints, skin, blood, and the brain.

It's All Connected

Every organ and system in the body is interconnected. Blood supplies life to every cell. Without a clean blood supply, cellular renewal cannot take place. Toxins absorbed into the bloodstream from the digestive system are often responsible for cellular deformation, which can lead to diseased organs and tissues.

The liver is an important organ that plays a critical role in detoxification. The liver protects our health and is responsible for vital functions such as helping to regulate blood sugar, energy, and hormone production. Liver enzymes convert toxins into nontoxic substances, which the kidneys eliminate. Both the liver and the kidneys need to function properly to keep the body free of poisonous substances. The liver processes food additives, preservatives and colorings, prescription drugs and over-the-counter medications, and environmental toxins. Once the liver becomes overburdened with toxic materials, the blood becomes toxic, and illness is inevitable.

To maximize liver function and bowel health, I recommend taking a purgative on day 6 of the detoxification and restoration week. Classic Ayurvedic texts recommend a purgative for type 2 diabetes, and medical research supports Ayurvedic theory. Purgatives eliminate toxins from the liver, gallbladder, and small intestine. This helps the body decongest bile, remove obstructions that inhibit metabolism and digestion, and function more efficiently. Studies show that purgatives designed according to Ayurvedic principles improve the strength of the metabolism, support proper elimination, remove unhealthy gut flora, improve sleep patterns, reduce heaviness in the abdomen, balance blood sugar, and reduce LDL and total cholesterol.

Purgation, however, is not recommended for everyone. Contraindications include rectal bleeding, ulcerative colitis, hemorrhoids, colon cancer, diarrhea, liver diseases, acid reflux, irritable bowel syndrome (IBS), fever, and infectious diseases. If you experience any of these conditions, skip drinking ghee or vegetable oil and the purgative on day 6.

The concept of detoxification goes back to antiquity. For thousands of years, Ayurveda practitioners have recognized the importance of digestive health for immunity, well-being, and longevity. Ayurveda has documented specific methods and treatments that detoxify the mind, body, and spirit, which are implemented in the detoxification and restoration week.

Detoxification Goals

- Burn fat
- Release toxins
- Improve digestion
- Reduce blood sugar

This detox will gently soften toxins and metabolic waste that obstruct the body's ability to digest foods and to eliminate waste properly from the body. The diet during this week is very similar to the 8-week elimination diet. Be sure to avoid white flour in any form, sugar, junk food, processed foods and meats, pesticides, chemicals, and preservatives. The detoxification diet also includes a delicious split mung bean and rice dish called kitchari and ingesting small amounts of ghee or oil. Having a daily massage, sipping warm water, taking herbs before and after meals, and taking a purgative on day 6 are also included. Plan your week so that day 6 is a rest day. Do the purgative on a day when you do not have to go to work, do chores, or have other commitments. The body needs to rest and focus on healing to receive the full benefits of the purgative. If that means continuing the elimination diet for a few more days to get day 6 to land on the right day, please do so.

Detoxification Program Structure

1. Eat a mostly kitchari diet on days 1–5.
2. Consume small amounts of oil on days 1–5.
3. Do bodywork treatments on days 1–5.
4. Take herbs before and after meals on days 1–5.
5. Sip warm water on days 1–7.
6. Take a purgative on day 6.
7. Eat light on days 6–7.

Detoxification Meal Plan

The meal plan includes deeply nourishing foods to help you clear toxins out of your body. Avoid alcohol, caffeine, food additives, colorings, preservatives, and refined and processed foods. The foods consumed during this period are warm and soupy. While the base of the meals is kitchari, you can add vegetables, grains, and other foods on your list to the kitchari base for more variety. But try to stick to a mostly kitchari diet for the first 5 days. Kitchari is a traditional Ayurvedic food used for detoxification, and it is essential during the 1-week detoxification and restoration. The combination of grains, beans, and herbs will vary depending on your constitution, but kitchari is beneficial for all.

Split yellow mung beans *(Vigna radiata)* are hulled and dried. They are much more digestible than whole or sprouted mung beans. Most people find split yellow mung beans easier on the digestive system than bigger beans, as they cause less gas. If you have difficulty digesting beans, try soaking the beans overnight before cooking. Soaking the beans removes compounds and indigestible sugars that can cause gas. Another advantage of soaking is that it reduces the cooking time. Just place the beans in a bowl with enough purified water to cover them by a couple of inches and soak overnight. In the morning, drain and rinse the beans before cooking.

If you soak the beans and still have difficulty digesting the kitchari, try adding a pinch of hing (asafetida) to the recipe. Hing is a powerful digestive agent that helps food move through the digestive tract. It dispels intestinal gas, relieves cramping, and reduces bloating. Hing also nourishes the intestinal flora and strengthens the digestive fire. When the digestive fire is robust, we can digest more difficult foods, such as beans.

Barley *(Hordeum vulgare)* is a cereal grain that is part of the kitchari recipe. Barley comes in several forms, including hulled or groats, hull-less, grits, flakes, pearls, quick, and flour. The whole, hulled form (also known as barley groats or Scotch barley) is the healthiest because only the tough, outer hull is removed, leaving the fiber and nutrients in the whole grain. Whole, hulled barley is not widely available but may be found in natural/whole food stores. Pearl barley is the most common, and, because it has been processed to remove the natural bran coating, it cooks faster and is less chewy.

Cumin, coriander, and fennel (CCF) is a popular formulation of culinary herbs in Ayurveda. CCF has been used throughout Ayurvedic history to remove metabolic waste and optimize digestion. Cumin helps remove toxins and clear mucus from the digestive tract. It kindles the digestive fire, relieving sluggish metabolism, diarrhea, intestinal spasms, and vomiting. Outside the digestive system, cumin reduces uterine inflammation.

Coriander stokes the digestive fire and prepares the liver for healthy digestion. Coriander is astringent, so it reduces excess kapha, mucus, and heaviness. Its cleansing action removes parasites from the body. Coriander is also a mild diuretic that cleanses and supports the urinary system. It has many benefits in alleviating type 2 diabetes.

Fennel helps reduce indigestion related to weak digestive strength. It alleviates abdominal pain, cramps, gas, and intestinal spasms. Fennel is cooling, so it doesn't aggravate pitta while it promotes the digestive fire. To prevent heartburn and reduce sugar cravings, simply chew a few seeds of fennel after meals.

Fenugreek is another culinary herb commonly used in Indian cuisine. The seed is used in curries as a digestion-promoting spice. Fenugreek is a mild laxative, which encourages the downward flow of energy in the pelvis. It reduces cholesterol and is suitable for convalescence, reproductive health, and the nervous system.

The combination of herbs, split yellow mung beans, and barley make kitchari ideal for healing the digestive system, increasing the metabolism, and balancing blood sugar. The beans are high in protein and fiber, packed with antioxidants, and rich in potassium, magnesium, and other nutrients. The barley adds fiber and balances blood glucose. And the herbs work to optimize the power of digestion and heal the digestive system. Not only that, kitchari tastes delicious!

Take your time to enjoy the aromas and flavors of kitchari. You can make a big pot and eat it throughout the day. Ayurveda, however, does not recommend eating leftovers, so make a fresh pot daily. I prefer to make kitchari on the stovetop, but you can also use a rice cooker, slow cooker, or pressure cooker.

Burning Fat

Fat is the body's endurance and blood-sugar-stabilizing fuel. Each morning, you will drink small, increasing amounts of melted ghee or vegetable oil and eat a simple diet to stimulate your metabolism and burn off fat-soluble toxins. Toxins such as preservatives, dioxin, pollutants, pesticides, and other damaging chemicals are stored in our fat cells. When we burn off fat, we remove the toxins that reside within it. Ghee and oil soften the gastrointestinal tract and create a cleansing action within the body, allowing us to gently remove toxins with the purgative without injuring the tissues where the toxins reside. If you have high cholesterol or are vegan, please use the recommended vegetable oil rather than ghee.

Reasons to Use Ghee

1. Ghee helps the body switch to fat-burning mode, which assists in weight loss.
2. Ghee can permeate the cell membrane and pull toxins from the tissues in the body without injuring them.
3. Ghee contains butyric acid, a fatty acid that feeds the beneficial bacteria in your gut, supporting a healthy microbiome.
4. Ghee is an excellent carrier; it delivers the therapeutic compounds from the medicinal herbs and spices in the kitchari recipe to the deep tissues of the body.
5. The butyric acid found in ghee supports the immune system by increasing the production of killer T-cells.
6. Research has shown that negative emotions have a biochemical form and

that ghee removes these toxic emotions as it cleanses the body.

7. Ghee stabilizes blood-sugar spikes and crashes.
8. Ghee decreases inflammation in the intestinal wall.
9. Ghee is high in conjugated linoleic acid (CLA), which improves insulin resistance and fights cancer.

Ghee is clarified, meaning it has the milk solids and water removed, leaving the pure essence of butter. Organic, unsalted, and cultured butter (preferably from grass-fed cows) is best for making ghee. Ready-made ghee is also available in some supermarkets and natural food stores, should you wish to purchase it. To check the quality of store-bought ghee, flip the jar over and examine the bottom—the ghee should be clear without any sediment.

MAKING GHEE AT HOME

Use a deep saucepan to allow for the foam to rise and to keep it from spilling over.

Ingredients:
- 1 pound unsalted butter, cut into 1-inch cubes (see note above)

Instructions:

1. Melt butter in a deep saucepan over medium-low heat and slowly bring it to a simmer, stirring occasionally for about 20 to 30 minutes. As the water cooks out of the butter, steam will rise. After the water is expelled, you will see foam rising from the gently simmering butter. Keep the butter slowly simmering without scraping the foam.
2. As the butter slowly simmers, the foam subsides and the milk solids begin to fall to the bottom of the pan. You may have to reduce the heat to low to keep the ghee from burning. Keep gently simmering without stirring until the ghee is transparent and you can see sediment on the bottom of the pan.
3. Remove the pan from the heat. Set aside for about 10 minutes or until it has cooled and the solids have settled. Line a fine mesh strainer with cheesecloth and pour the liquid ghee through the strainer into a mason jar. Discard the solids and cheesecloth. Set ghee aside to cool overnight and then cap and label the jar.
4. Ghee can be stored at room temperature; it does not need to be refrigerated. Always use a clean, dry spoon or utensil to scoop ghee to prevent it from turning rancid.

Bodywork Treatments

Dry Skin Massage: Days 1–2

Garshana or dry skin massage is an Ayurvedic technique used for detoxification of the skin, lymphatic system, and fat cells. Traditional Ayurvedic garshana uses silk gloves. Today, people may use a natural bristled brush or textured washcloth to get many of the same effects.

The health benefits of dry skin massage are many. It encourages lymphatic drainage, promotes blood flow, and stimulates the immune system to detoxify the body. Dry skin massage exfoliates and removes dead skin cells, loosens fat pockets that contribute to cellulite, and creates fresher, healthier skin. Dry skin massage is not only detoxifying, but it is also restorative. It calms the nerves, promotes self-love, and provides deep relaxation. And if that weren't enough, it also feels great!

Dry skin massage is a vital part of days 1–2 of the detoxification. The skin is the body's largest organ, and it is responsible for removing one-quarter of the waste from the body. Dry skin massage is a quick, inexpensive, and effective way to help the body detoxify.

The ideal time to give yourself a dry skin massage is in the morning before a shower. Please give yourself plenty of time to relax and enjoy it. Make sure you are warm, relaxed, and in a comfortable spot. After you finish the massage, rinse off the impurities in the shower.

Be aware that there are contraindications for dry skin massage. If your skin is insensitive, e.g., if you experience diabetic neuropathy, be very careful not to apply too much pressure. You can injure yourself. People who have sensitive skin, inflamed skin, cracked or broken skin, high blood pressure, eczema, psoriasis, rashes, slow-healing wounds, or skin infections should avoid dry skin massage.

Choosing a Dry Skin Massage Tool

Make sure the tool you choose for dry skin massage is soft and not too abrasive. If you would like to go the traditional route, you can use special Ayurvedic silk gloves called garshana gloves. You can also choose a dry skin brush with a long handle for hard-to-reach places. Brushes come in a variety of natural and synthetic fibers. Natural fibers are generally softer and made of animal hair. Brushes with synthetic fibers may be a little stiffer, but they are suitable for people opposed to using animal products. You may also use a dry, textured washcloth. Be very careful not to apply too much pressure, as you could injure your skin.

Dry Skin Massage Instructions

1. Begin by massaging the soles of your feet in circular motions. Work your way around to the tops of your feet and progress to your ankles, calves, and thighs.
2. Use circular strokes on the stomach and joints (shoulders, elbows, knees, wrists, hips, and ankles) and long sweeping strokes on the arms and legs. The stroke should always be toward your heart; this helps drain the lymph back to your heart.
3. To aid digestion, massage the abdomen with circular, clockwise motions, following the natural flow of the colon.
4. Stroke over to the hips, continuing the upward, circular motions. In the upper chest area, apply gentle pressure as the skin there is sensitive.
5. Apply light pressure where the skin is thin, such as the underarms, and harder pressure where the skin is thicker, such as the soles of the feet.
6. Brush from the forearms toward the upper arms. Once you reach the shoulders, begin brushing downwards toward the heart. Repeat this on your back.
7. From the neck area, brush down. From your buttocks and lower back, brush up.
8. Incorporate a 5-minute dry skin massage ritual into your daily routine for the first 2 days of the detoxification program.

Abhyanga *(Loving Embrace Self-Massage)*: Days 3–5

Abhyanga is a vital part of days 3–5 of the detoxification week. Massaging the body with oil loosens deep-seated toxins that reside in the joints, muscles, and fat tissues of the body. An abhyanga self-massage lubricates the joints, increases circulation, stimulates the organs, assists in the elimination of impurities, moves lymph, increases stamina, calms the nerves, promotes self-love, and provides deep relaxation and restoration.

It is best to do abhyanga first thing in the morning. Give yourself plenty of time to relax and enjoy the massage. Make sure you are warm and comfortable. After you finish abhyanga, you can put on an old robe or sweats that you don't mind getting oily. Be mindful of oily feet. They can be quite slippery, so put on some socks or slippers.

Abhyanga Self-Massage Instructions

- Begin by running some hot water over the bottle to warm the oil recommended for your dosha (listed below).
- Pour warm oil into your palm and work into your scalp. Using your

fingertips, vigorously massage your head and scalp with small circular strokes, as if you are shampooing.
- If you don't want to oil your head, you can massage your head with dry hands.
- Move to your face and ears, massaging more gently in a circular motion.
- Place a little more oil in your hands and, with an open hand, apply pressure to the sides and back of the neck.
- Vigorously rub your arms, using a circular motion at the shoulders and elbows and back-and-forth motions on the long bones of the upper arms and forearms.
- Make a circle with your pointer finger and thumb and massage your wrists in a circular motion. Massage the palms of your hands in a circular motion. Then make a circle with your pointer finger and thumb and massage each finger, using more pressure as you move toward the body.
- Massage your chest and stomach, using a gentle circular clockwise motion and a straight up-and-down motion over the breastbone and hips.
- Apply oil to both hands, reach around to the back and spine, and massage yourself as well as you can without straining.
- Use circular motions over your hips and vigorously rub your legs as you did your arms, applying more pressure to your thighs. Use a circular motion at the knees and ankles and back-and-forth motions on the shins and the backs of the legs.
- After massaging your legs, spend extra time on your feet. With the palm of your hand, massage vigorously back and forth over the soles and tops of the feet.
- Keep a thin film of oil on your body.
- Allow the oil to soak into your skin for 10 to 15 minutes, and then rinse it off in the shower.

Herbs Before and After Meals: Days 1–5

Taking herbs before meals will increase your body's digestive enzymes and improve digestion. It is also helpful for flatulence, malabsorption, nausea, and indigestion. Taking herbs after meals will increase your metabolism and decrease metabolic waste.

- **Before meals**: Chew ¼ teaspoon of freshly grated ginger with a squeeze of lemon (vata/kapha) or lime (pitta). Consume 15 minutes before meals. You can grate enough ginger to last 5 days and store it in the fridge.
- **After meals**: Chew a pinch of dry-roasted whole fennel seeds. To dry roast fennel seeds, place seeds in a pan over medium heat, stirring

frequently, for 2 to 3 minutes or until golden brown. Store in an airtight container.

Sipping Warm Water: Days 1–7

Sip warm-to-hot water throughout the day. Hot water softens the intestinal tract, moves lymph, and hydrates cells more effectively than cold water. To create this softening, cleansing atmosphere in the body, sip boiled warm-to-hot water throughout the day. The water must be plain to have a detoxifying and hydrating effect. It can be tempting to add a lemon, but please just sip plain, warm water without anything added. When we add juice to water, it creates more work for the body. Because the body must metabolize the juice to absorb the water, try to stick with plain water. Your goal is to consume at least half your body weight in ounces per day. For example, if you weigh 200 pounds, your goal is to drink 100 ounces of warm water daily. The easiest way to accomplish this is to boil 100 ounces, allow it to cool for a few minutes, and then transfer the water into a thermos or two and carry it with you to drink throughout the day.

Purgative on Day 6

The purgative removes toxins from the digestive system, including the liver, gallbladder, and pancreas. Purgation clears the channels so that energy can flow freely. Drinking small amounts of ghee or vegetable oil leading up to the purgation softens toxins and metabolic waste, so harmful materials can easily be removed from the body without injuring it.

Purgation affects everyone differently. After you take the purgative, you may have several bowel movements. There may be periods of discomfort associated with the release of toxins. During this time, your body is undergoing a deep cellular cleansing. If you feel nauseated, sip on a little ginger tea. By the afternoon, the bowel movements should be complete, and you will feel light, energized, and refreshed. It is essential to continue to rest for the remainder of the day. When you start to feel hunger, eat a light meal, such as a watery vegetable soup, and avoid napping.

Choosing Your Purgative

Choose your purgative based on your digestive symptoms and elimination:
- If you experience heartburn, acidic indigestion, nausea, or loose stools, take 1 tablespoon of psyllium husks in 8 ounces of warm water.
- If you have regular bowel movements without gas, bloating, loose stools, or constipation, take 1 tablespoon of triphala in 3 ounces of warm water.
- If you have heaviness, gas, bloating, or hard or constipated stools, take 2

tablespoons of castor oil.

1-Week Detox and Restoration for Vata

Basic Detox Supplies:
- Organic ghee or organic, cold-pressed sesame oil
- Kitchari ingredients (see recipe that follows)
- Dry skin brush, garshana gloves, or washcloth
- Abhyanga massage oil (organic, cold-pressed sesame oil)
- Purgative (see page 161)

KITCHARI RECIPE FOR VATA

Makes: 2 servings
Ingredients:
- ¼ cup yellow split dried mung beans
- ¾ cup barley
- 1 tablespoon ghee (see page 164) or sesame oil
- ¼ teaspoon mustard seeds
- ⅛ teaspoon hing/asafetida
- ½ teaspoon whole cumin seeds, ground
- ½ teaspoon whole coriander seeds, ground
- ½ teaspoon whole fennel seeds, ground
- ½ teaspoon fenugreek powder
- ½ teaspoon turmeric powder
- 4 cups water

Instructions:
1. Combine beans and barley in a colander. Rinse well and set aside to drain.
2. Heat ghee in a large saucepan over medium heat. Add mustard seeds and heat until they pop. Add hing, cumin, coriander, fennel, fenugreek, and turmeric and stir well.
3. Stir in beans, barley, and water. Increase heat to high and bring to a boil. Reduce heat to low. Simmer for 45 minutes, stirring occasionally, or until the water has been absorbed and the consistency is like soupy porridge. For variety, add 2 cups of chopped vegetables in the last 10 minutes of cooking.

7-Day Schedule for Vata

Day 1: Drink 1 tablespoon of melted ghee or sesame oil, and then wait at least 30 minutes before eating. Eat kitchari and other meals (no snacks) from foods on the vata list. Walk after meals. Sip warm water throughout the day. Do a dry skin massage followed by a warm shower. Practice breathing exercises, yoga, and meditation; rest and relax; and go to bed early.

Day 2: Drink 4 teaspoons (1 tablespoon + 1 teaspoon) of melted ghee or sesame oil, and then wait at least 30 minutes before eating. Eat kitchari and other meals (no snacks) from foods on the vata list. Take herbs before and after meals. Walk after meals. Sip warm water throughout the day. Do a dry skin massage followed by a warm shower. Practice breathing exercises, yoga, and meditation; rest and relax; and go to bed early.

Day 3: Drink 5 teaspoons (1 tablespoon + 2 teaspoons) of melted ghee or sesame oil, and then wait at least 30 minutes before eating. Eat kitchari and other meals (no snacks) from foods on the vata list. Take herbs before and after meals. Walk after meals. Sip warm water throughout the day. Do an abhyanga warm oil massage followed by a warm shower. Practice breathing exercises, yoga, and meditation; rest and relax; and go to bed early.

Day 4: Drink 2 tablespoons of melted ghee or sesame oil, and then wait at least 30 minutes before eating. Eat kitchari and other meals (no snacks) from foods on the vata list. Take herbs before and after meals. Walk after meals. Sip warm water throughout the day. Do an abhyanga warm oil massage followed by a warm shower. Practice breathing exercises, yoga, and meditation; rest and relax; and go to bed early.

Day 5: Drink 7 teaspoons (2 tablespoons + 1 teaspoon) of melted ghee or sesame oil, and then wait at least 30 minutes before eating. Eat kitchari and other meals (no snacks) from foods on the vata list. Take herbs before and after meals. Walk after meals. Sip warm water throughout the day. Do an abhyanga warm oil massage followed by a warm shower. Practice breathing exercises, yoga, and meditation; rest and relax; and go to bed early.

Note: If nausea occurs after taking the ghee or sesame oil, sip ½ to 1 cup of warm-to-hot water with fresh lemon juice and grated ginger root or try mixing the ghee with warm organic nut milk. If nausea persists, do not increase the dose of ghee the next day. Take the same amount or less!

Day 6 (Purgative): Contraindications for the purgative include rectal bleeding, ulcerative colitis, hemorrhoids, colon cancer, diarrhea, liver diseases, acid reflux, IBS, fever, and infectious diseases. If you do not have any of these conditions, you can proceed with the purgative.

Early in the morning, before you eat or drink anything, take a hot Epsom salt bath or hot shower and then ingest the appropriate purgative (see page 161). Everybody is different, but it may take 1 to 2 hours for the laxative effect to begin. Then you may have several bowel movements over the next few hours. During this time, your body undergoes a deep cellular cleansing as it removes deep-seated toxins that were interfering with your metabolism. Afterward, you will feel light, energized, and refreshed. But it is essential to continue to rest for the remainder of the day. When you start to feel hunger, eat a light meal. Sip warm water throughout the day. Do not take a nap.

Day 7: Eat light! Whatever you eat, make sure you don't overeat. The purgative pulled out some of your digestive fire along with the toxins. Work slowly to rebuild your digestive strength. Think of your digestive fire as a small flame; if you put a big log on it, the log will extinguish the fire. The foods you choose to eat could either feed the fire or suffocate it. Big heavy meals act like a big log, and small meals like kindling. Try to eat bland food that gradually increases in complexity. Heavy meals will cause gastric upset. Eat slowly and eat smaller portions; you'll discover you don't need a lot of food to feel full. Take the time to appreciate how good food tastes. Chew slowly and in a relaxed space.

1-Week Detox and Restoration for Pitta

Basic Detox Supplies:
- Organic ghee or flaxseed oil
- Kitchari ingredients (see recipe that follows)
- Garshana gloves, dry skin brush, or washcloth
- Abhyanga massage oil (organic sunflower oil)
- Purgative (see page 161)

KITCHARI RECIPE FOR PITTA

Makes 2 servings

Ingredients:
- ¾ cup yellow split dried mung beans
- ¼ cup barley
- 1 tablespoon ghee or extra-virgin sunflower oil
- ¼ teaspoon whole cumin seeds, ground
- 1 teaspoon whole coriander seeds, ground
- 1 teaspoon whole fennel seeds, ground
- ½ teaspoon fenugreek powder
- ½ teaspoon turmeric powder
- 4 cups water

Instructions:
1. Combine beans and barley in a colander. Rinse well and set aside to drain.
2. Heat ghee in a large saucepan over medium heat. Add cumin, coriander, fennel, fenugreek, and turmeric and stir well.
3. Stir in beans, barley, and water. Increase heat to high and bring to a boil. Reduce heat to low. Simmer for 45 minutes or until the water has been

absorbed and the consistency is similar to soupy porridge. For variety, add 2 cups of chopped vegetables in the last 10 minutes of cooking.

7-Day Schedule for Pitta

Day 1: Drink 1 teaspoon of melted ghee or flaxseed oil, and then wait at least 30 minutes before eating. Eat kitchari and other meals (no snacks) from foods on the pitta list. Take herbs before and after meals. Walk after meals. Sip warm water throughout the day. Do a dry skin massage followed by a warm shower. Practice breathing exercises, yoga, and meditation; rest and relax; and go to bed early.

Day 2: Drink 2 teaspoons of melted ghee or flaxseed oil, and then wait at least 30 minutes before eating. Eat kitchari and other meals (no snacks) from foods on the pitta list. Take herbs before and after meals. Walk after meals. Sip warm water throughout the day. Do a dry skin massage followed by a warm shower. Practice breathing exercises, yoga, and meditation; rest and relax; and go to bed early.

Day 3: Drink 1 tablespoon of melted ghee or flaxseed oil, and then wait at least 30 minutes before eating. Eat kitchari and other meals (no snacks) from foods on the pitta list. Take herbs before and after meals. Walk after meals. Sip warm water throughout the day. Do an abhyanga warm oil massage followed by a warm shower. Practice breathing exercises, yoga, and meditation; rest and relax; and go to bed early.

Day 4: Drink 4 teaspoons (1 tablespoon + 1 teaspoon) of melted ghee or flaxseed oil, and then wait at least 30 minutes before eating. Eat kitchari and other meals (no snacks) from foods on the pitta list. Take herbs before and after meals. Walk after meals. Sip warm water throughout the day. Do an abhyanga warm oil massage followed by a warm shower. Practice breathing exercises, yoga, and meditation; rest and relax; and go to bed early.

Day 5: Drink 5 teaspoons (1 tablespoon + 2 teaspoons) of melted ghee or flaxseed oil, and then wait at least 30 minutes before eating. Eat kitchari and other meals (no snacks) from foods on the pitta list. Take herbs before and after meals. Walk after meals. Sip warm water throughout the day. Do an abhyanga warm oil massage followed by a warm shower. Practice breathing exercises, yoga, and meditation; rest and relax; and go to bed early.

Note: If nausea occurs after taking the ghee or sesame oil, sip ½ to 1 cup of warm-to-hot water with fresh lemon juice and grated ginger root or try mixing the ghee with warm organic nut milk. If nausea persists, do not increase the dose of oil the next day. Take the same amount or less!

Day 6 (Purgative): Contraindications for the purgative include rectal bleeding, ulcerative colitis, hemorrhoids, colon cancer, diarrhea, liver diseases, acid reflux, IBS, fever, and infectious diseases. If you do not have any of these conditions, you can proceed with the purgative.

Early in the morning, before you eat or drink anything, take a hot Epsom salt bath or hot shower and then ingest the appropriate purgative (see page 161). Everybody is different, but it may take 1 to 2 hours for the laxative effect to begin. Then you may have several bowel movements over the next few hours. During this time, your body undergoes a deep cellular cleansing as it removes deep-seated toxins that were interfering with your metabolism. Afterward, you will feel light, energized, and refreshed. But it is essential to continue to rest for the remainder of the day. When you start to feel hunger, eat a light meal. Sip warm water throughout the day. Do not take a nap.

Day 7: Eat light! Whatever you eat, make sure you don't overeat. The purgative pulled out some of your digestive fire along with the toxins. Work slowly to rebuild your digestive strength. Think of your digestive fire as a small flame; if you put a big log on it, the log will extinguish the fire. The foods you choose to eat could either feed the fire or suffocate it. Big heavy meals act like a big log, and small meals like kindling. Try to eat bland food that gradually increases in complexity. Heavy meals will cause gastric upset. Eat slowly and eat smaller portions; you'll discover you don't need a lot of food to feel full. Take the time to appreciate how good food tastes. Chew slowly and in a relaxed space.

1-Week Detox and Restoration for Kapha

Basic Detox Supplies:
- Organic ghee or flaxseed oil
- Kitchari ingredients (see recipe that follows)
- Garshana gloves, dry skin brush, or washcloth
- Abhyanga massage oil (organic sunflower oil)
- Purgative (see page 161)

KITCHARI RECIPE FOR KAPHA
Makes: 2 servings
Ingredients:
- ½ cup yellow split dried mung beans
- ½ cup barley
- 1 tablespoon ghee or extra-virgin sunflower oil
- 1 teaspoon mustard seeds
- ½ teaspoon whole cumin seeds, ground
- ½ teaspoon whole coriander seeds, ground
- ½ teaspoon whole fennel seeds, ground
- ½ teaspoon fenugreek powder
- ½ teaspoon turmeric powder

- 4 cups water

Instructions:

1. Combine beans and barley in a colander. Rinse well and set aside to drain.
2. Heat ghee in a large saucepan over medium heat. Add mustard seeds and heat until they pop. Add cumin, coriander, fennel, fenugreek, and turmeric and stir well.
3. Stir in beans, barley, and water. Increase heat to high and bring to a boil. Reduce heat to low. Simmer for 45 minutes or until the water has been absorbed and the consistency is similar to soupy porridge. For variety, add 2 cups of chopped vegetables in the last 10 minutes of cooking.

7-Day Schedule for Kapha

Day 1: Drink 1/2 teaspoon of melted ghee or flaxseed oil, and then wait at least 30 minutes before eating. Eat kitchari and other meals (no snacks) from foods on the kapha list. Take herbs before and after meals. Walk after meals. Sip warm water throughout the day. Do a dry skin massage followed by a warm shower. Practice breathing exercises, yoga, and meditation; rest and relax; and go to bed early.

Day 2: Drink 1 teaspoon of melted ghee or flaxseed oil, and then wait at least 30 minutes before eating. Eat kitchari and other meals (no snacks) from foods on the kapha list. Take herbs before and after meals. Walk after meals. Sip warm water throughout the day. Do a dry skin massage followed by a warm shower. Practice breathing exercises, yoga, and meditation; rest and relax; and go to bed early.

Day 3: Drink 1 1/2 teaspoons of melted ghee or flaxseed oil, and then wait at least 30 minutes before eating. Eat kitchari and other meals (no snacks) from foods on the kapha list. Take herbs before and after meals. Walk after meals. Sip warm water throughout the day. Do an abhyanga warm oil massage followed by a warm shower. Practice breathing exercises, yoga, and meditation; rest and relax; and go to bed early.

Day 4: Drink 2 teaspoons of melted ghee or flaxseed oil, and then wait at least 30 minutes before eating. Eat kitchari and other meals (no snacks) from foods on the kapha list. Take herbs before and after meals. Walk after meals. Sip warm water throughout the day. Do an abhyanga warm oil massage followed by a warm shower. Practice breathing exercises, yoga, and meditation; rest and relax; and go to bed early.

Day 5: Drink 2 1/2 teaspoons of melted ghee or flaxseed oil, and then wait at least 30 minutes before eating. Eat kitchari and other meals (no snacks) from foods on the kapha list. Take herbs before and after meals. Walk after meals. Sip warm water throughout the day. Do an abhyanga warm oil massage followed by a warm shower. Practice breathing exercises, yoga, and meditation; rest and relax; and go to bed early.

Note: If nausea occurs after taking the ghee or sesame oil, sip ½ to 1 cup of warm-to-hot water with fresh lemon juice and grated ginger root or try mixing the ghee with warm organic nut milk. If nausea persists, do not increase the dose of oil the next day. Take the same amount or less!

Day 6 (Purgative): Contraindications for the purgative include rectal bleeding, ulcerative colitis, hemorrhoids, colon cancer, diarrhea, liver diseases, acid reflux, IBS, fever, and infectious diseases. If you do not have any of these conditions, you can proceed with the purgative.

Early in the morning, before you eat or drink anything, take a hot Epsom salt bath or hot shower and then ingest the appropriate purgative (see page 161). Everybody is different, but it may take 1 to 2 hours for the laxative effect to begin. Then you may have several bowel movements over the next few hours. During this time, your body undergoes a deep cellular cleansing as it removes deep-seated toxins that were interfering with your metabolism. Afterward, you will feel light, energized, and refreshed. But it is essential to continue to rest for the remainder of the day. When you start to feel hunger, eat a light meal. Sip warm water throughout the day. Do not take a nap.

Day 7: Eat light! Whatever you eat, make sure you don't overeat. The purgative pulled out some of your digestive fire along with the toxins. Work slowly to rebuild your digestive strength. Think of your digestive fire as a small flame; if you put a big log on it, the log will extinguish the fire. The foods you choose to eat could either feed the fire or suffocate it. Big heavy meals act like a big log, and small meals like kindling. Try to eat bland food that gradually increases in complexity. Heavy meals will cause gastric upset. Eat slowly and eat smaller portions; you'll discover you don't need a lot of food to feel full. Take the time to appreciate how good food tastes. Chew slowly and in a relaxed space.

CHAPTER 10

The 12-Week Program: 3-Week Rebuilding and Reintroduction of Foods

Congratulations! You made it to the third and final part of the program! In the first part, you removed foods from your diet that are not compatible with your constitution. You used clinically proven herbs, daily walks, a regular exercise program, a relaxation routine, sleep optimization, and other lifestyle changes to improve type 2 diabetes.

The daily exercise and relaxation practices used to maintain a balanced state throughout the program should continue to be a part of your lifestyle. The exercise program helped you build muscle, maintain an active lifestyle, and metabolize glucose more efficiently. The breathwork, meditation, and relaxation practices kept you calm and reduced stress-induced blood-sugar spikes. Exercise and relaxation work together and are excellent tools to restore the mind, body, and spirit. Please continue to use what you learned in the first part of the program for daily strengthening, rejuvenation, and longevity. The key to health is continual rejuvenation.

In the second part of the program, you performed a home Ayurvedic detoxification called panchakarma. Throughout this process, you removed toxins that were interfering with your metabolism. Relieved of the work of digesting incompatible foods that upset digestion, metabolism, and elimination, your body could focus on repairing and healing itself. You restored yourself with a daily massage that eliminated toxic substances from the deep tissues. You have now detoxified and renewed yourself holistically. Your digestive system is running optimally with less inflammation and fewer unhealthy bacteria.

Detoxification is part of the Ayurvedic lifestyle. We are constantly exposed to environmental and dietary toxins, so it is important to regularly detoxify. Ayurveda advises us to detoxify with the change of the seasons. The winter and summer solstices and the fall and spring equinoxes are the ideal times to perform the home Ayurvedic detoxification.

Reintroduction of Foods

Goals:

- Create an individualized diet to support your unique constitution.
- Introduce new foods into the diet.

The return to one's everyday diet should be gradual. Introducing too many heavy, hard-to-digest foods at one time can be strenuous on the digestive system, throwing off your digestive fire and reversing all your hard work. It is essential to maintain a diet free of sugar, processed foods, and additives. Continue with a diet high in fiber, low-glycemic fruits and vegetables, whole grains, and good-quality, lean protein.

In the third part of the program, you will introduce more foods that are compatible with your constitution. You may find that some foods are easy to metabolize and can be a part of your diet. In contrast, others may raise your blood glucose too high and should be kept out of your diet. Your goal is to determine which foods you can safely include in *your* long-term diet and which foods should stay out. All the foods you enjoyed on your food list should continue to be part of your daily diet.

When reintroducing foods, keep a food journal to monitor your symptoms. Please keep track of all your changes in symptoms, blood glucose levels, digestion, elimination, etc., in the Blood Sugar and Food Journal (see page 186).

Testing your blood glucose after meals is an essential part of the reintroduction process. This will help reduce hyperglycemia and the risk of developing long-term type 2 diabetes complications. It is best to test your blood glucose 2 hours after reintroducing a new food, so pay attention to the time when you start your meal. For example, if you want to reintroduce sweet potatoes, and you sit down to eat at 6:00 p.m., check your blood glucose at 8:00 p.m. After the meal, don't eat anything else before testing your blood glucose. When you check your blood glucose at 8:00 p.m., write down your results and note what factors may have affected them, such as the quantity of food, other foods you ate with the meal, and your level of activity and stress. Test results may also vary depending on your age, gender, health history, and the method used for the test. Take a close look at your blood glucose record to see if your level is too high as you introduce each new food. If your blood glucose is above 140 mg/dL 2 hours after your meal, try the food again the next day to see if your blood glucose is still above 140 mg/dL 2 hours after eating it. If so, it may not be a food that you want to include in your diet. Do this with each new food for the next 3 weeks. Keep track of the foods in your Blood Sugar and Food Journal so that you remember which foods to include and which foods to eliminate.

Out-of-range blood glucose numbers can leave you upset, confused, frustrated, angry, or sad. It's easy to use the numbers to judge yourself, so it is important to remember that tracking your blood glucose level is simply a way to know how well your care plan is working and which foods your body is properly digesting. Testing post-meal blood glucose will help you discover how your body responds to specific foods after eating a meal. As you digest the food in your stomach, blood glucose levels rise sharply. In response, your pancreas releases insulin to help remove this sugar from your blood and transport it into your muscles and other tissues, where it is used for energy. Within 2 hours of eating, your insulin and blood glucose levels should return to normal. If your blood glucose levels remain high, there is a problem in the process.

The reintroduction of foods works well for determining how well your body is digesting foods. If there is a spike in your blood sugar, you now know which food is causing a reaction. Post-meal glucose spikes can be uniquely damaging to health, so minimizing them is a priority. It is crucial to monitor how your body reacts to individual foods.

There is simply no one-size-fits-all eating plan that works for everyone. Different people can have very different glycemic reactions to the same foods, and the impact of lifestyle choices and other individual factors are challenging to measure with traditional tools. Regular glucose monitoring 2 hours after meals provides objective information about how *your* food and lifestyle choices affect *your* glucose levels. In this part of the program, you will create an individualized diet to support your unique constitution based on your body's blood glucose response.

When reintroducing foods, start with the lightest, easiest foods to digest such as fruits and vegetables and work your way up to more difficult-to-digest foods. Introducing heavy foods too soon could compromise the strength of your digestion, so gradually work your way up. The specific foods introduced each week will depend on your constitution. Fruits and vegetables for each constitution are introduced the first week. The second week may include dairy or beans or various grains. The third week includes meats, seafood, and dairy. If you want to include foods that are not specifically recommended for your constitution, please include them in the week they are recommended.

Vata 3-Week Food Reintroduction Schedule

- Week 1—apricots, bananas, dates, figs, mango, melons, peaches, papaya,

rice (all kinds), raisins (soaked), sweet potatoes, pumpkin
- Week 2—dairy (butter, buttermilk, hard and soft cheese, cottage cheese, cow's milk, goat's milk, sour cream, diluted and spiced yogurt), wheat
- Week 3—meats and seafood (beef, buffalo, duck, fish, salmon, sardines, shrimp, tuna)

Pitta 3-Week Food Reintroduction Schedule
- Week 1—apricots, couscous, dates, figs, mangos, melons, papaya, plums, potatoes (sweet, white), pumpkin, prunes, raisins, rice (basmati), white beans
- Week 2—dairy (cottage cheese, cow's milk, goat milk, goat cheese), wheat
- Week 3—buffalo, fish, shrimp, venison

Kapha 3-Week Food Reintroduction Schedule
- Week 1—apricots, figs, peaches, pears, persimmons, potatoes (white), raisins
- Week 2—corn flour, couscous, granola, polenta, rice (basmati), rye, spelt, wheat, wheat bran, white beans
- Week 3—buttermilk, cottage cheese, fish, goat cheese, goat milk, shrimp

CHAPTER 11

CLOSING THOUGHTS

You have made it through the 12-week program! It's time to toast yourself with a nice glass of warm water! Making the transition into the Ayurvedic lifestyle for type 2 diabetes is no easy task. I'm sure there were days when you did not feel like getting up at the recommended wake time or eating the foods on your list or going for a walk after a meal, but you did it! And at this point, I'm going to ask you to take a good look at who you were at the beginning of the program and compare it to who you are now. What's different about you? Are you satisfied with the changes? Did you meet your health goals? Has your sense of well-being changed? Have you noticed the effects different foods have on your constitution? Have your tastes and cravings changed?

Ayurveda is transformative medicine. When you follow its principles, noticeable changes occur. At first, these shifts may feel subtle. Digestive disturbances such as gas, bloating, and indigestion start to clear. But after a couple of weeks, your body composition begins to change; fat burns, and muscles build. Muscle development creates more energy. Metabolic waste melts away as your digestive power increases. As your body purifies itself, energy increases, and the organs can channel this energy into healing and repair. Organ functioning is no longer compromised by toxic burdens, and the doshas can flow freely throughout the body. But this 12-week journey has been more than a physical transformation. It's been an illuminating experience that you felt at your core. The relaxation practices created space and clarity within your mind. As negative thought patterns dissolved, your reaction to stress became calmer and your overall disposition became more grounded and peaceful.

Over the course of the last 12 weeks, you have gotten to know your constitution and have explored your strengths and imbalances. It takes courage to look at yourself through the Ayurvedic lens and shift your perspective on health and wellness. Ayurveda has supported the health of millions of people for thousands of years. Yet, it is unfamiliar to most Western healthcare providers and their patients. When you chose to try Ayurveda, you chose a conscious, experience-based medical system, and through this program, you rejuvenated yourself. Ayurveda is now part of your daily life, and once you go Ayurveda, you can never go back!

It takes passion to commit to an Ayurvedic lifestyle and change your daily routine, try new foods, commit to an exercise program, explore meditation, and complete a detox. I'm sure many of these practices were new to you, and I hope they stay with you. Throughout this 12-week journey, you have persevered because of your passion to take control of your health. It is this passion that will give you the momentum to continue your wellness journey. Take the time throughout each day to connect to your breath. Stay grounded in your constitution, remember who you are, and use the Ayurvedic tools to bring yourself back into balance. You now know how to find serenity amongst the chaos. Be mindful in your daily practices. Take the time to slowly chew your foods and enjoy all the rich flavors and tastes. Treat yourself to a detox with the solstices and equinoxes. Give yourself a break at the end of the day to enjoy the transition into twilight. Let yourself settle into your breath to transport your mind and body into relaxation. Follow the natural order of life, and it will bring you to happiness. Pay attention to signs and symptoms when you are feeling out of balance and tap into your wellspring of inner wisdom and healing potential. If you give your mind and body the proper resources to thrive, it will! Take what you have learned throughout this program to help support your friends, family, and community.

I am continually amazed at the balance Ayurveda has created in my own life. It truly is lifestyle medicine. The simple rituals from the Vedic sciences have allowed me to become aware of the present, tune in with the rhythms of nature, and become established within my constitution. Ayurveda is a functional medicine that any person can benefit from, and I practice it because I know it changes lives. Thank you for trusting me as your guide down the Ayurvedic path.

Your Ayurvedic journey doesn't have to end here, however. I encourage you to go deeper. In the Resources section of this book, you will find a list of some of my most beloved and respected teachers. If you are interested in a professional consultation or panchakarma treatment, please see pages 183–184.

Consultations with Jackie Christensen, PhD: Practice Ayurveda

By using a mix of ancient wisdom and modern science, we will identify your unique mind-body type and develop a holistic treatment plan just for you. Your naturopathic and Ayurvedic treatment can be as in-depth as you choose, and we offer a wide variety of packages, bodywork treatments, detox plans, group programs, and more.
Website: www.practiceayurveda.com
Phone: 831-818-6660
Email: jackie@practiceayurveda.com

Ayurvedic Healing

Highly individualized panchakarma clinic based on the needs of the individual depending on the Ayurvedic constitutional type, doshic imbalances, age, digestive strength, immune status, and many other factors.
Website: https://www.ayurvedichealing.net
Phone: 831-462-3776
Email: info@ayurvedichealing.net

Ayurveda World

Ayurveda World provides a wide range of herbal remedies and specializes in compounded herbal formulas and hand-made Ayurvedic products, such as herbal teas, massage oils, and tinctures. All of their products use sustainably sourced and made from organic ingredients whenever possible.
Website: https://ayurveda-world-herb-store.square.site
Phone: 408-847-4385
Email: ayurveda-world@mountmadonna.org

BMI Calculator

Body mass index (BMI) is a measure of body fat based on height and weight that applies to adult men and women. Calculate your BMI with the National Institute of Health's BMI calculator.
Website: https://www.nhlbi.nih.gov/health/educational/lose_wt/BMI/bmicalc.htm

Kaya Kalpa Wellness Center
Kaya Kalpa means "rejuvenation of body and spirit," and their professionally trained practitioners are dedicated to your well-being. They offer a variety of Ayurvedic therapies, traditional massage, and other body therapies.
Phone: 408-846-4078
Email: kayakalpa@mountmadonna.org

Lotus Holistic Health Institute
Lotus Holistic Health Institute is an Ayurvedic day spa that provides panchakarma services, consultations, and workshops. Treatments are structured so that anyone can enjoy the full panchakarma program or select from one of the luxurious bodywork therapies.
Website: lotusayurveda.com
Phone: 1-831-566-0735

National Ayurvedic Medical Association (NAMA)
The National Ayurvedic Medical Association represents the Ayurvedic profession in the United States. The purpose of the association is to provide leadership within the Ayurvedic profession and to promote a positive vision for Ayurveda and its holistic approach to health and wellness.
Website: www.ayurvedanama.org
Phone: 213-628-6291

Mount Madonna Institute of Ayurveda
Since 1978, Mount Madonna has provided theoretical and practical professional education and training in classical systems of Yoga, Ayurveda, and Community. Each school emphasizes self-learning, service, and continuing lifelong learning, as well as teaching the ethical and professional standards necessary for developing high-level, meaningful careers.
Website: www.mountmadonnainstitute.org
Phone: 408-846-4060
Email: admissions@mountmadonnainstitute.org

Mount Madonna Institute of Ayurveda Clinic

Ayurveda consultations are provided by their highly qualified Ayurvedic faculty practitioners. Initial consultations consist of a brief explanation of Ayurveda and a detailed history, including focused Ayurvedic evaluation, mind-body type, and imbalances. Treatment plans may include Ayurvedic diet, lifestyle routine, herbs, yoga, pranayama, and meditation.

Phone: 408-846-4060
Email: consultations@mountmadonnainstitute.org

Maharishi Ayurveda Products International

Serve your health needs with Ayurvedic herbal products, including silk garshana gloves.

Website: https://www.mapi.com
Phone: 800-255-8332
Email: CustomerService@mapi.com

Yoga Journal

Yoga Journal is a source for in-depth yoga pose instruction, yoga sequences for beginners to advanced practitioners, and guided audio meditations to keep your day stress free.

Website: www.yogajournal.com

Blood Sugar and Food Journal

With each meal, you can reintroduce one new food. Write down each food you reintroduce in the "Food Introduced" column. In the "Additional Foods & Beverages Consumed" column, write any other foods and drinks you consumed with the new food you reintroduced. In the "Activity After Eating" column, write down what you did during the 2 hours after the meal. For example, if you walked, exercised, worked, or watched TV, write it in the column. Blood sugar test results may vary depending on stress level and level of activity. Two hours after consumption of the new food, test your blood sugar and record the result in the "Blood Sugar 2 Hours After Reintroduction of Food" column. If your blood sugar is above 140 mg/dL 2 hours after your meal, try the food again the next day to see if your blood sugar is still above 140 mg/dL 2 hours after eating it. If so, it may not be a food that you want to include in your diet. Do this with each new food for the next 3 weeks.

Week 1, Day 1

Vata Foods to Reintroduce: apricots, bananas, dates, figs, mango, melons, peaches, papaya, rice (all kinds), raisins (soaked), sweet potatoes, pumpkin
Pitta Foods to Reintroduce: apricots, couscous, dates, figs, mangos, melons, papaya, plums, potatoes (sweet, white), pumpkin, prunes, raisins, rice (basmati), white beans
Kapha Foods to Reintroduce: apricots, figs, peaches, pears, persimmons, potatoes (white), raisins

Meal	Food Introduced	Additional Foods & Beverages Consumed	Activity After Eating	Blood Sugar 2 Hours After Reintroduction of Food
Breakfast				
Lunch				
Dinner				

Week 1, Day 2

Meal	Food Introduced	Additional Foods & Beverages Consumed	Activity After Eating	Blood Sugar 2 Hours After Reintroduction of Food
Breakfast				
Lunch				
Dinner				

Week 1, Day 3

Meal	Food Introduced	Additional Foods & Beverages Consumed	Activity After Eating	Blood Sugar 2 Hours After Reintroduction of Food
Breakfast				
Lunch				
Dinner				

Week 1, Day 4

Meal	Food Introduced	Additional Foods & Beverages Consumed	Activity After Eating	Blood Sugar 2 Hours After Reintroduction of Food
Breakfast				
Lunch				
Dinner				

Week 1, Day 5

Meal	Food Introduced	Additional Foods & Beverages Consumed	Activity After Eating	Blood Sugar 2 Hours After Reintroduction of Food
Breakfast				
Lunch				
Dinner				

Week 1, Day 6

Meal	Food Introduced	Additional Foods & Beverages Consumed	Activity After Eating	Blood Sugar 2 Hours After Reintroduction of Food
Breakfast				
Lunch				
Dinner				

Week 1, Day 7

Meal	Food Introduced	Additional Foods & Beverages Consumed	Activity After Eating	Blood Sugar 2 Hours After Reintroduction of Food
Breakfast				
Lunch				
Dinner				

Week 2, Day 1

Vata Foods to Reintroduce: dairy (butter, buttermilk, hard and soft cheese, cottage cheese, cow's milk, goat's milk, sour cream, diluted and spiced yogurt), wheat
Pitta Foods to Reintroduce: dairy (cottage cheese, cow's milk, goat milk, goat cheese), wheat
Kapha Foods to Reintroduce: corn flour, couscous, granola, polenta, rice (basmati), rye, spelt, wheat, wheat bran, white beans

Meal	Food Introduced	Additional Foods & Beverages Consumed	Activity After Eating	Blood Sugar 2 Hours After Reintroduction of Food
Breakfast				
Lunch				
Dinner				

Week 2, Day 2

Meal	Food Introduced	Additional Foods & Beverages Consumed	Activity After Eating	Blood Sugar 2 Hours After Reintroduction of Food
Breakfast				
Lunch				
Dinner				

Week 2, Day 3

Meal	Food Introduced	Additional Foods & Beverages Consumed	Activity After Eating	Blood Sugar 2 Hours After Reintroduction of Food
Breakfast				
Lunch				
Dinner				

Week 2, Day 4

Meal	Food Introduced	Additional Foods & Beverages Consumed	Activity After Eating	Blood Sugar 2 Hours After Reintroduction of Food
Breakfast				
Lunch				
Dinner				

Week 2, Day 5

Meal	Food Introduced	Additional Foods & Beverages Consumed	Activity After Eating	Blood Sugar 2 Hours After Reintroduction of Food
Breakfast				
Lunch				
Dinner				

Week 2, Day 6

Meal	Food Introduced	Additional Foods & Beverages Consumed	Activity After Eating	Blood Sugar 2 Hours After Reintroduction of Food
Breakfast				
Lunch				
Dinner				

Week 2, Day 7

Meal	Food Introduced	Additional Foods & Beverages Consumed	Activity After Eating	Blood Sugar 2 Hours After Reintroduction of Food
Breakfast				
Lunch				
Dinner				

Week 3, Day 1

Vata Foods to Reintroduce: meats and seafood (beef, buffalo, duck, fish, salmon, sardines, shrimp, tuna)
Pitta Foods to Reintroduce: buffalo, fish, shrimp, venison
Kapha Foods to Reintroduce: buttermilk, cottage cheese, fish, goat cheese, goat milk, shrimp

Meal	Food Introduced	Additional Foods & Beverages Consumed	Activity After Eating	Blood Sugar 2 Hours After Reintroduction of Food
Breakfast				
Lunch				
Dinner				

Week 3, Day 2

Meal	Food Introduced	Additional Foods & Beverages Consumed	Activity After Eating	Blood Sugar 2 Hours After Reintroduction of Food
Breakfast				
Lunch				
Dinner				

Week 3, Day 3

Meal	Food Introduced	Additional Foods & Beverages Consumed	Activity After Eating	Blood Sugar 2 Hours After Reintroduction of Food
Breakfast				
Lunch				
Dinner				

Week 3, Day 4

Meal	Food Introduced	Additional Foods & Beverages Consumed	Activity After Eating	Blood Sugar 2 Hours After Reintroduction of Food
Breakfast				
Lunch				
Dinner				

Week 3, Day 5

Meal	Food Introduced	Additional Foods & Beverages Consumed	Activity After Eating	Blood Sugar 2 Hours After Reintroduction of Food
Breakfast				
Lunch				
Dinner				

Week 3, Day 6

Meal	Food Introduced	Additional Foods & Beverages Consumed	Activity After Eating	Blood Sugar 2 Hours After Reintroduction of Food
Breakfast				
Lunch				
Dinner				

Week 3, Day 7

Meal	Food Introduced	Additional Foods & Beverages Consumed	Activity After Eating	Blood Sugar 2 Hours After Reintroduction of Food
Breakfast				
Lunch				
Dinner				

ACKNOWLEDGMENTS

Writing this book was a dharmic journey in which I found myself vastly supported by my Ayurvedic teachers and writing community. Deep gratitude and thanks to my great teachers and inspirers—without them, I would not be the person I am today. Dr. Vasant Lad for his wisdom and contributitions to the Ayurvedic community, which helped me dive into the subtle aspects of this book. I am immensely grateful to Vaidyas Suhas G. Kshirsagar, Manisha Kshirsagar, Cynthia Copple, John Douillard, and Rucha Kelkar for your kindness and willingness to give this book your love and attention. Your lessons and teachings of the Vedic sciences have helped me understand the nature of my destination.

Mount Madonna Institute instructors and administration for creating a vibrant community for me to explore, learn, and grow. Your love for Ayurveda is truly exceptional.

I am indebted to the many researchers and scientists who worked to publish the studies that provided the undeniable credibility for many of the recommendations in this book.

To my agent Linda Konner, who believed in this book and advocated for me from the beginning; to Elizabeth Hudson, my editor, for providing clarity and thoughtful insight; to Mary Glenn and Keith Pfeffer for supporting the process and steering the ship; and to all my clients, who trust me as their guide down the Ayurvedic path for type 2 diabetes—my gratitude. As a teacher, I learn so much from my students.

Jackie Christensen

Jackie Christensen is an expert in the field of Ayurveda healing, and my thanks go to her for expanding this exceptional book to include my recipes. Linda Konner's experience and ability to spot a winning manuscript at first blush is exceptional. I'm grateful to be a writer in her fold. The publishing world is challenging and rapidly changing, and the team at Humanix—Mary Glenn and Keith Pfeffer—are pivoting with the times and continue to put great books into the hands of readers. I'm blessed to have a partner, Gary McLaughlin, who embraces the rhythms of our separate creative projects.

Pat Crocker

Jackie Christensen

Jackie Christensen, PhD, knows how to open people's hearts and minds while providing pragmatic, easy-to-follow instructions that can change lives. Jackie received her doctorate in natural medicine and holds a master's degree in Ayurveda. In addition, she is a certified nutritional consultant, master herbalist, and holistic health practitioner.

Jackie has served on the faculty of many respected colleges. She has hosted international study-abroad programs as well as local workshops, classes, and conferences. Jackie is an internationally recognized educator in natural health, herbology, and Ayurveda. She has appeared on the highly rated PBS program *American Health Journal*, and she contributes to How to Cure. Jackie currently has a private practice in Santa Cruz, California, where she specializes in type 2 diabetes therapies.

Visit her at practiceayurveda.com.

Pat Crocker

Pat has been a student of healing food and herbal wisdom for many decades. During the 1990s, she led wild herb walks from Riversong Cabin, her 150-year-old home (at the time) in rural Grey County. Her "teaching garden" provided the herbs for her workshops on preparing simple healing tinctures, salves, and teas.

Since that time, Pat has written 23 cookbooks, including *The Healing Herbs Cookbook*, *The Juicing Bible* (over 800,000 copies in print, translated into over 10 languages), and her newest books, *The Herbalist's Kitchen*, and *Cooking with Cannabis*.

Pat is a professional Home Economist (BAA, BEd).

Visit her at patcrocker.com.

A

Ayurveda, overview of, 1–3

B

barley
Amaranth Breakfast Bowl, 134–135
Barley and Spinach Scramble, 76–77
Barley Polenta, 84–85
barley tea, 98–99, 125–126, 155–156
cooking instructions, 21–22
kitchari, 163, 170, 172, 174–175
Mung Bean and Barley Stew, 79–80
Mushroom Barley Chicken Stew, 137–138
overview of, 20–22
Warm Barley Breakfast Bowl, 77
bitter green vegetables, 26
bitter melon
kapha dosage, 156
overview of, 23
pitta dosage, 126
vata dosage, 99
blood sugar
barley and, 20–22
goals for, 56
journal, 57, 186–196
monitoring, 55–57
mung beans and, 26
oversaturation, 13–14, 16
stress and, 38, 46
virechana purification, 51–53
"weak tissue" and, 15–16
bowel movements, 159–160, 169
brain
breathwork and, 43
exercise and, 33–34
breathwork
brain function and, 43
kapha program, 148
pitta program, 120–121
stress reduction with, 42–44
vata program, 92–93

C

cardiovascular exercise. *See also*
exercise.
benefits of, 31
boot-camp exercises, 153–154

cycling, 152–153
examples of, 32, 124
fartlek, 152
hill repeats, 152
journal, 155
swimming, 124
yoga as, 154
cinnamon
Amaranth Breakfast Bowl, 134–135
barley tea, 98–99, 125–126, 155–156
Breakfast Bowl with Golden Milk, 106
Chia Seed Pudding, 77–78
Golden Coconut Milk, 104
Overnight Oat-Apple Bowl, 78–79
overview of, 25
constitution
discovering, 64–65
overview of, 10–11
quiz, 66–70
sleep and, 36
walking and, 29–30
cumin, coriander, and fennel (CCF),
100, 163

D

daily schedules
establishing, 61
kapha program, 144
pitta program, 116
vata program, 88–89
detox and restoration
abhyanga massage, 167–168
Ayurveda and, 161
body interconnectivity, 161
bowel movements, 159–160
bowel toxemia, 160
dry skin massage, 166–167
fat-burning, 164–165
ghee, 164–165
goals, 162
gut permeability, 160
health problems, 160
herbs at mealtime, 168–169
kapha program, 174–176
kitchari, 162–164, 170, 172, 174–175
liver and, 161
meal plan, 162–164
panchakarma treatment, 50–53

parasites, 160–161
pitta program, 172–174
program structure, 162
purgatives, 161, 169–170
reasons to detoxify, 158–159
toxicity signs, 159–161
vata program, 170–172
virechana purification, 51–53
water, 169

E

exercise. *See also* cardiovascular
    exercise; resistance training;
    walking; yoga.
  brain and, 33–34
  cycling, 152–153
  injuries, 63–64
  intensity monitoring, 62
  interval workouts, 151–152
  journal, 98, 155
  kapha program, 151–155
  maximum heart rate (MHR), 62–63
  pilates, 123–124
  pitta program, 123–125
  program formulation, 31–33
  RICE formula, 63–64
  sedentary time, 34–35
  vata program, 96–98
  weightlifting, 123

F

fennel
  after meals, 168
  benefits of, 163
  flavor profile, 100
  Cauliflower Fennel Soup, 141–142
  Pitta Vegetable-Mung Bean Pots with
    Seed Crust, 111
fenugreek, 23–24, 163–164

G

ghee
  benefits of, 164–165
  Green Egg Frittata, 78
  Mung Bean and Barley Stew, 79
  recipe, 165
  storage, 165
ginger
  before meals, 168
  Ginger Lemonade, 75
  overview of, 24–25

H

herbal therapies
  ayaskriti formulation, 49–50
  chandraprabha vati formulation, 49
  gurmar/madhuharini/sardunika
    (*Gymnema sylvestre*), 46
  neem (*Azadirachta indica*), 45–46
  pharmaceutical drugs and, 44–45
  triphala formulation, 48
  tulsi (*Ocimum sanctum L.*), 46–47

J

jackfruit
  overview of, 22–23
  Spiraled Zucchini with Jackfruit and
    Cilantro Pesto, 112
journal pages
  biometric journal, 57
  food reintroduction, 186–196
  kapha relaxation, 150
  kapha exercise, 155
  pitta relaxation, 122
  pitta exercise, 125
  vata relaxation, 95
  vata exercise, 98

K

kapha
  aggravations, 9
  constitution and, 64
  daily routine and, 61
  detox and restoration schedule,
    174–176
  dominant elements, 8
  kapha-type diabetes, 16–17
  lifestyle, 13, 15, 144–155
  overview of, 2–3, 8–10
  reintroduction schedule, 180
  six tastes and, 19–20
  sleep and, 36
kapha basic recipes
  Aloe Basil Margarita, 131
  Fire-Roasted Marinara, 132
  Grilled Salsa, 132–133
  Spinach Pesto, 131–132
kapha breakfast recipes
  Amaranth Breakfast Bowl, 134–135
  Artichoke and Sundried Tomato
    Scramble, 133–134
  Blueberry Power Bars, 134
  Fruit Salad, 135

Quick and Easy Quinoa Bowl,
    135–136
kapha constitution and elimination diet
    astringent tastes, 128
    awareness meditation, 148–149
    bitter tastes, 127–128
    breathwork, 148
    daily schedule, 144
    exercise program, 151–155
    food lists, 128–131
    lifestyle enhancement, 144–145
    pungent tastes, 127
    relaxation practice, 145–150
    resistance training, 151, 153
    responsibilities, 8–9
    sleep optimization, 143–144
    supplement schedule, 155–157
    yoga practice, 145–147, 154
kapha dinner recipes
    Cauliflower Fennel Soup, 141–142
    Cauliflower Rice with Lemon, Kale,
        and Parsley, 139
    Chickpea Vegetable Soup, 142–143
    Kapha Vegetable Mung Bean Pots
        with Seed Crust, 141
    Mint-Cilantro Chutney, 140
    Mung Bean Patties, 139–140
    Roasted Garlic and Mung Beans, 143
kapha lunch recipes
    Beet and Carrot Spirals with Roasted
        Vegetables, 138–139
    Chicken and Sautéed Brussels
        Sprouts, 136
    Chicken Fajita Bowl, 136–137
    Eggplant and Turkey with Pesto, 138
    Fajita Seasoning, 137
    Mushroom Barley Chicken Stew,
        137–138
kitchari
    ingredient overview, 162–164
    kapha recipe, 174–175
    pitta recipe, 172–173
    vata recipe, 170

M
massage
    abhyanga massage, 167–168
    dry skin massage, 166–167
meditation
    awareness meditation, 148–149
    stress reduction with, 40–42

tratak meditation, 121
    yoga nidra meditation, 93–94
metabolic waste
    accumulation of, 13–14, 16, 158
    gut permeability and, 160
    nervous system and, 18
    parasites and, 160–161
    virechana purification, 51–53
mindfulness
    meditation, 148–149
    mindful eating, 60–61
    yoga and, 39
mung beans
    Kapha Vegetable Mung Bean Pots
        with Seed Crust, 141
    kitchari, 163, 170, 172–173, 174–175
    Mung Bean and Barley Stew, 79–80
    Mung Bean and Coconut Curry,
        83–84
    Mung Bean Dip, 104–105
    Mung Bean Patties, 139–140
    overview of, 26
    Pitta Vegetable-Mung Bean Pots with
        Seed Crust, 111
    Roasted Garlic and Mung Beans, 143

N
neem (*Azadirachta indica*)
    kapha dosage, 156
    overview of, 45–46
    pitta dosage, 126

P
pitta
    aggravations, 6–7
    constitution, 64
    daily routine and, 61
    detox and restoration schedule,
        172–174
    dominant elements, 6
    inflammation and, 7–8
    overview of, 2–3, 5–8
    physical traits, 5–6
    pitta-type diabetes, 17
    reintroduction schedule, 180
    responsibilities, 6
    sleep and, 36
pitta basic recipes
    Cilantro Pesto, 105
    Golden Coconut Milk, 104
    Mung Bean Dip, 104–105

pitta breakfast recipes
  Breakfast Bowl with Golden Milk, 106
  Broccoli Mushroom Scramble, 107
  Coconut-Berry Overnight Oatmeal
    Bowl, 105–106
  Pancakes and Fruit, 107–108
  Zucchini Kale Scramble, 108
pitta constitution and elimination diet
  astringent tastes and, 100–101
  bitter tastes and, 100–101
  breathwork, 120–121
  cardiovascular exercise, 124–125
  daily schedule, 116–117
  exercise program, 123–125
  food lists, 101–104
  lifestyle enhancement, 116–117
  progressive muscle relaxation,
    115–116
  relaxation practice, 117–122
  resistance training, 123–124
  sleep, 114–115
  supplement schedule, 125–126
  tratak meditation, 121
  yoga practice, 117–120
pitta dinner recipes
  Black Bean Bowl, 113–114
  Cauliflower Lime Rice, 114
  Creamy Broccoli Soup, 113
  Creamy Red Lentil Veggie Soup, 112
  Spiraled Zucchini with Jackfruit and
    Cilantro Pesto, 112
pitta lunch recipes
  Chicken Deluxe Salad, 109
  Pitta Vegetable-Mung Bean Pots with
    Seed Crust, 111
  Turkey with Parsnips and Green
    Beans, 110
  Vegetable Coins with Chicken and
    Avocado Drizzle, 108–109
  Zucchini Turkey Burgers, 109–110
purgation
  contraindications, 161
  function of, 51, 161
  kapha program, 176
  pitta program, 173
  scheduling, 162
  selection, 169–170
  vata program, 171
  virechana purification, 51

R
reintroduction schedule, 178–180
relaxation
  kapha program, 145–150
  pitta program, 117–122
  progressive muscle relaxation,
    115–116
  sleep optimization and, 87
  vata program, 89–95
  yoga and, 39
resistance training. See also exercise.
  benefits of, 28, 31
  kapha program, 151, 153
  pitta program, 123–124
  vata program, 96–97

S
sleep
  breathwork and, 43–44
  importance of, 35–36
  insomnia, 36, 86–88
  kapha program, 143–144
  napping, 36–37
  pitta program, 114–115
  vata program, 86–88
stress
  blood sugar and, 38, 46
  breathwork and, 42–44
  cortisol and, 87
  meditation and, 40–42
  physical response to, 38
  type 2 diabetes and, 37–39
  yoga and, 39–40
supplements
  barley tea, 98–99, 125–126, 155–156
  bitter melon, 99, 126, 156
  Gymnema sylvestre, 99, 126, 156
  kapha, 155–157
  neem, 126, 156–157
  pitta program, 125–126
  triphala, 99, 126, 156
  tulsi, 99, 156
  vata program, 98–99

T
toxicity. See detox and restoration.
triphala formulation
  benefits of, 48
  kapha program 156
  pitta program, 126
  vata program, 99

tulsi (*Ocimum sanctum L.*)
  kapha program 156
  overview of, 46–47
  vata program, 99
turmeric, 24

U
urination, 14, 49–50

V
vata
  aggravations, 4–5
  constitution and, 64
  daily routine and, 61
  detox and restoration schedule,
    170–172, 174–176
  dominant elements, 4
  overview of, 2–3, 3–5
  physical traits, 3
  reintroduction schedule, 179–180
  responsibilities, 4
  sleep and, 36
  vata–type diabetes, 17–18
vata basic recipes
  Artichoke Tahini, 75
  Ginger Lemonade, 75
  Pesto, 75–76
  Roasted Garlic, 76
vata breakfast recipes
  Barley and Spinach Scramble, 76–77
  Chia Seed Pudding, 77–78
  Green Egg Frittata, 78
  Overnight Oat-Apple Bowl, 78–79
  Warm Barley Breakfast Bowl, 77
vata constitution and elimination diet
  daily relaxation journal, 95
  daily schedule, 88–89
  exercise program, 96–98
  food lists, 72–74
  goals for, 71
  lifestyle enhancement, 89
  relaxation practice, 89–95
  resistance training, 96–97
  sleep optimization, 86–88
  sour tastes, 71–72
  supplement schedule, 98–99
  walking after meals, 97–98
vata dinner recipes
  Barley Polenta, 84–85
  Mung Bean and Coconut Curry,
    83–84

Quinoa Bowl with Lentils and
  Vegetables, 83
Red Lentil Pasta, 86
Spaghetti Squash with Kale and
  Garlic, 85
vata lunch recipes
  Chicken Taco Salad with Avocado
    Dressing, 80–81
  Chicken with Bok Choy, 81
  Green Chili Turkey Burgers, 82
  Mung Bean and Barley Stew, 79–80
  Thai Red Curry Chicken, 81–82

W
walking. *See also* exercise.
  after meals, 61–62, 97–98
  benefits of, 28–30
  constitution and, 29–30
  intensity monitoring, 62
  vata program, 97–98

Y
yoga. *See also* exercise.
  Alternate Nostril Breathing Practice,
    92–93
  Cat/Cow Pose, 118
  Cobra Pose (*Bhujangasana*), 147
  Corpse Pose (*Savasana*), 92, 119–120,
    147
  Extended-Leg Forward Bend
    (*Paschimatanasana*), 118, 146–147
  Happy Baby Pose (*Ananda Balasana*),
    90
  kapha program, 154
  Kneeling Forward Bend
    (*Mandukasana*), 145–146
  Legs on a Chair, 90–91
  Legs Up the Wall, 90–92
  Reclined, Supported Bound Angle
    Pose (*Baddha Konasana*), 118–119
  Seated Spinal Twist (*Vakrasana*), 146
  stress reduction with, 39–40
  Wind Relieving Pose (*Pavana*
    Muktasana), 89–90, 119
  Yoga Nidra Meditation Practice,
    93–94

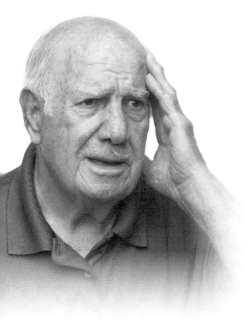

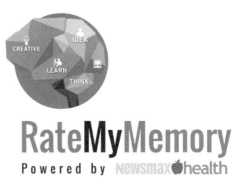

RateMyMemory
Powered by newsmax❤health

Normal Forgetfulness?
Something More Serious?

You forget things — names of people, where you parked your car, the place you put an important document, and so much more. Some experts tell you to dismiss these episodes.

"Not so fast," say the editors of Newsmax Health, and publishers of *The Mind Health Report.*

The experts at Newsmax Health say that most age-related memory issues are normal but sometimes can be a warning sign of future cognitive decline.

Now Newsmax Health has created the online **RateMyMemory Test** — allowing you to easily assess your memory strength in just a matter of minutes.

It's time to begin your journey of making sure your brain stays healthy and young! **It takes just 2 minutes!**

Test Your Memory Today:
MemoryRate.com/Type

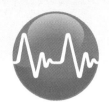 Simple **Heart Test**

Powered by Newsmaxhealth.com

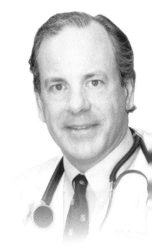

FACT:

▸ Nearly half of those who die from heart attacks each year never showed prior symptoms of heart disease.

▸ If you suffer cardiac arrest outside of a hospital, you have just a 7% chance of survival.

Don't be caught off guard. Know your risk now.

TAKE THE TEST NOW ...

Renowned cardiologist **Dr. Chauncey Crandall** has partnered with **Newsmaxhealth.com** to create a simple, easy-to-complete, online test that will help you understand your heart attack risk factors. Dr. Crandall is the author of the #1 best-seller *The Simple Heart Cure: The 90-Day Program to Stop and Reverse Heart Disease.*

Take Dr. Crandall's Simple Heart Test — it takes just 2 minutes or less to complete — it could save your life!

Discover your risk now.

- Where you score on our unique heart disease risk scale
- Which of your lifestyle habits really protect your heart
- The true role your height and weight play in heart attack risk
- Little-known conditions that impact heart health
- Plus much more!

SimpleHeartTest.com/Type